M000160093

Copyright 2020 by Michelle Robinson -All rights reserved.

No part of this publication may be reproduced, distributed, or transmitted in any form or by any means, including photocopying, recording, or other electronic or mechanical methods, without the prior written permission of the publisher, except in the case of brief quotations embodied in reviews and certain other non-commercial uses permitted by copyright law.

This Book is provided with the sole purpose of providing relevant information on a specific topic for which every reasonable effort has been made to ensure that it is both accurate and reasonable. Nevertheless, by purchasing this Book you consent to the fact that the author, as well as the publisher, are in no way experts on the topics contained herein, regardless of any claims as such that may be made within. It is recommended that you always consult a professional prior to undertaking any of the advice or techniques discussed within.This is a legally binding declaration that is considered both valid and fair by both the Committee of Publishers Association and the American Bar Association and should be considered as legally binding within the United States.

CONTENTS

Superfoods Stir Fry Recipes

Allergy labels: SF – Soy Free, GF – Gluten Free, DF – Dairy Free, EF – Egg Free, V - Vegan, NF – Nut Free

Superfoods Stir Fry Marinade

This marinade has 100% Superfoods ingredients and it's great with any meat or fish and even veggies. Sesame oil and sesame seeds are Superfoods, just like ginger, garlic, scallions, black pepper and red hot chili flakes. I personally don't use soy at all and I replaced soy sauce with fish sauce but you can use soy sauce if you want. Red wine is also Superfood rich in anthocyanidins, quercetin and resveratrol.

- 3 tbsp. fish sauce - optional soy sauce
- 2 tsp. sesame oil
- 1 tsp. freshly grated ginger
- 1 garlic clove, diced
- 1/4 cup red wine or chicken broth or both

Optional:
- 1 Tbsp. arrowroot flour - if you want your stir fry thicker
- 1/4 cup chopped scallions
- 1 tsp. chili flakes (adjust for heat)
- 1/2 tsp. ground black pepper

Korean Spicy Stir Fry Marinade

- 3 tbsp. fish sauce - optional soy sauce
- 1 tsp. sesame oil
- 1 tsp. freshly grated ginger
- 1 garlic clove, diced
- 1 tsp. chili flakes or powder (adjust for heat)

Pork, Bok Choy & Celery Stir Fry

Serves 2 - Allergies: SF, GF, DF, EF, NF
- 10 o.z. Lean Pork Tenderloin
- 2 cups Bok Choy
- 1 cup chopped celery
- 1 tsp coconut oil

Marinade pork in a Superfoods marinade. Stir fry drained pork in coconut oil and when it's no longer pink add celery and stir fry for 1 more minute. Add bok choy and stir fry for a minute longer and then add the rest of the marinade and stir fry for one more minute.

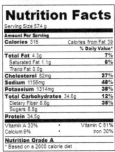

Lemon Chicken Stir Fry

Serves 3-4
Ingredients - Allergies: SF, GF, DF, EF, NF
- 1 lemon
- 1/2 cup chicken broth
- 3 tbsp. fish sauce
- 2 teaspoons arrowroot flour
- 1 tbsp.oil
- 1 pound boneless, skinless chicken breasts, trimmed and cut into 1-inch pieces
- 10 ounces mushrooms, halved or quartered
- 2 cups snow peas, stems and strings removed
- 1 bunch scallions, cut into 1-inch pieces, white and green parts divided
- 1 tbsp. chopped garlic

Instructions

Grate 1 tsp. lemon zest. Juice the lemon and mix 3 tbsp. of the juice with broth, fish sauce and arrowroot flour in a small bowl.

Heat oil in a skillet over high heat. Add chicken and cook, stirring occasionally, until just cooked through. Transfer to a plate. Add mushrooms to the pan and cook until the mushrooms are tender. Add snow peas, garlic, scallion whites and the lemon zest. Cook, stirring, around 30 seconds. Add the broth to the pan and cook, stirring, 2 to 3 minutes. Add scallion greens and the chicken and any accumulated juices and stir.

Pan seared Brussels sprouts

Serves 2

Ingredients - Allergies: SF, GF, DF, EF, NF
- 6 oz. cubed pork
- 2 tbsp.oil
- 1 pound Brussels sprouts, halved
- 1/2 large onion, chopped
- Salt and ground black pepper

Instructions

Cook pork in a skillet over high heat. Remove to a plate and chop. In same pan with pork fat, add coconut oil over high heat. Add onions and Brussels sprouts and cook, stirring occasionally, until sprouts are golden brown. Season with salt and pepper, to taste, and put pork back into pan. Serve immediately.

Beef and Broccoli Stir Fry

Serves 2 - Allergies: SF, GF, DF, EF, NF
- 10 o.z. Beef
- 2 cups Broccoli
- 1 tsp coconut oil

Marinade beef in a Superfoods marinade. Stir fry drained beef in coconut oil and when it's no longer pink add broccoli and stir fry for 2 more minutes. Add the rest of the marinade and stir fry for a minute. Serve with brown rice or quinoa.

Nutrition Facts	
Serving Size 251 g	
Amount Per Serving	
Calories 342	Calories from Fat 124
	% Daily Value*
Total Fat 13.8g	**21%**
Saturated Fat 4.0g	**20%**
Trans Fat 0.0g	
Cholesterol 127mg	**42%**
Sodium 1024mg	**43%**
Potassium 884mg	**25%**
Total Carbohydrates 7.0g	**2%**
Dietary Fiber 2.4g	**10%**
Sugars 1.7g	
Protein 46.5g	
Vitamin A 11% •	Vitamin C 131%
Calcium 5% •	Iron 154%
Nutrition Grade A-	
* Based on a 2000 calorie diet	

Garbanzo Stir Fry

Serves 2
Ingredients - Allergies: SF, GF, DF, EF, V, NF
• 2 tbsp.oil • 1 tbsp. oregano • 1 tbsp. chopped basil • 1 clove garlic, crushed •
ground black pepper to taste • 2 cups cooked garbanzo beans
• 1 large zucchini, halved and sliced • 1/2 cup sliced mushrooms • 1 tbsp. chopped
cilantro • 1 tomato, chopped
Heat oil in a skillet over medium heat. Stir in oregano, basil, garlic and pepper. Add
the garbanzo beans and zucchini, stirring well to coat with oil and herbs. Cook for 10
minutes, stirring occasionally. Stir in mushrooms and cilantro; cook 10 minutes,
stirring occasionally. Place the chopped tomato on top of the mixture to steam.
Cover and cook 5 minutes more.

Thai Basil Chicken

Serves 1
Ingredients - Allergies: SF, GF, DF, NF
For the egg
• 1 egg
• 2 tbsp. of coconut oil for frying
Basil chicken
• 1 chicken breast (or any other cut of boneless chicken, about 200 grams)
• 5 cloves of garlic
• 4 Thai chilies
• 1 tbsp.oil for frying
• Fish sauce
• 1 handful of Thai holy basil leaves
Instructions
First, fry the egg.
Basil chicken
Cut the chicken into small pieces. Peel the garlic and chilies, and chop them fine. Add
basil leaves.
Add about 1 tbsp. of oil to the pan.
When the oil is hot, add the chilies and garlic. Stir fry for half a minute.
Toss in your chicken and keep stir frying. Add fish sauce.
Add basil into the pan, fold it into the chicken, and turn off the heat.

Shrimp with Snow Peas

Serves 4.

Ingredients - Allergies: SF, GF, DF, EF, NF

Marinade
- 2 teaspoons arrowroot flour
- 1 Tbsp red wine
- 1/2 tsp. salt

Stir Fry
- 1 pound shrimp, peeled and deveined
- 2 Tbspoil
- 1 Tbsp minced ginger
- 3 garlic cloves, sliced thinly
- 1/2 pound snow peas, strings removed
- 2 teaspoons fish sauce
- 1/4 cup chicken broth
- 4 green onions, white and light green parts, sliced diagonally
- 2 teaspoons dark roasted sesame oil

Instructions

Mix all the ingredients for the marinade in a bowl and then add the shrimp. Mix to coat. Let it marinade 15 minutes while you prepare the peas, ginger, and garlic. Add the coconut oil in the wok and let it get hot. Add the garlic and ginger and combine. Stir-fry for about 30 seconds.

Add the marinade to the wok, add the snow peas, fish sauce and chicken broth. Stir-fry until the shrimp turns pink. Add the green onions and stir-fry for one more minute. Turn off the heat and add the sesame oil. Toss once more and serve with steamed brown rice or soba gluten free noodles.

Pork and Green Beans Stir Fry

Serves 1 - Allergies: SF, GF, DF, EF, NF

- 6oz. of lean Pork
- 1 cup of Green Beans, snapped in half. Use as much veggies as you want or replace Green beans with Kale.
- 1 garlic clove, chopped
- 1/2 inch of peeled and chopped ginger
- Season with fish sauce.

Nutrition Facts	
Serving Size 285 g	
Amount Per Serving	
Calories 317	Calories from Fat 97
	% Daily Value*
Total Fat 10.8g	17%
Saturated Fat 2.7g	14%
Trans Fat 0.1g	
Cholesterol 124mg	41%
Sodium 104mg	4%
Potassium 946mg	27%
Total Carbohydrates 7.8g	3%
Dietary Fiber 3.7g	15%
Sugars 1.5g	
Protein 46.5g	
Vitamin A 15% •	Vitamin C 30%
Calcium 5% •	Iron 17%
Nutrition Grade A	
* Based on a 2000 calorie diet	

Cashew chicken

Serves 4

Ingredients - Allergies: SF, GF, DF, EF, NF
- 1 bunch scallions
- 1 pound skinless boneless chicken thighs
- 1/2 tsp. salt
- 1/4 tsp. black pepper
- 3 tbsp.oil
- 1 red bell pepper and 1 stalk of celery, chopped
- 4 garlic cloves, finely chopped
- 1 1/2 tbsp. finely chopped peeled fresh ginger
- 1/4 tsp. dried hot red-pepper flakes
- 3/4 cup chicken broth
- 1 1/2 tbsp. fish sauce
- 1 1/2 teaspoons arrowroot flour
- 1/2 cup salted roasted whole cashews

Instructions

Chop scallions and separate green and white parts. Pat chicken dry and cut into 3/4-inch pieces and season with salt and pepper. Heat a wok or a skillet over high heat. Add oil and then stir-fry chicken until cooked through, 3 to 4 minutes. Transfer to a plate. Add garlic, bell pepper, celery, ginger, red-pepper flakes, and scallion whites to wok and stir-fry until peppers are just tender, 4 to 5 minutes.

Mix together broth, fish sauce and arrowroot flour, then stir into vegetables in wok. Reduce heat and simmer, stirring occasionally, until thickened. Stir in cashews, scallion greens, and chicken along with any juices.

Bass Celery Tomato Bok Choy Stir Fry

Serves 2
Ingredients - Allergies: SF, GF, DF, EF
- 1/2 pound bass fillets • 1 cup Celery
- 1/2 cup sliced Tomatoes
- 1/2 cup sliced Bok Choy
- 1/2 cup sliced carrots and cucumbers
- 1 Tsp.oil *Instructions*

Marinade bass in a Superfoods marinade. Stir fry drained bass in coconut oil for few minutes, add all vegetables and stir fry for 2 more minutes. Add the rest of the marinade and stir fry for a minute. Serve with brown rice or quinoa.

Broccoli, Yellow Peppers & Beef Stir Fry

Serves 2
Ingredients - Allergies: SF, GF, DF, EF
- 1/2 pound beef • 1 cup Broccoli
- 1/2 cup sliced Yellow Peppers
- 1/2 cup chopped onions
- 1 Tbsp. sesame seeds
- 1 Tsp.oil *Instructions*

Marinade beef in a Superfoods marinade. Stir fry drained beef in coconut oil for few minutes, add all vegetables and stir fry for 2 more minutes. Add the rest of the marinade and stir fry for a minute. Serve with brown rice or quinoa.

Chinese Celery, Mushrooms & Fish Stir Fry

Serves 2
Ingredients - Allergies: SF, GF, DF, EF
- 1/2 pound fish fillets • 1 cup Chinese Celery
- 1 cup Mushrooms sliced in half
- 1/2 cup peppers sliced diagonally
- 1 Tsp.oil *Instructions*

Marinade fish in a Superfoods marinade. Stir fry drained fish in coconut oil for few minutes, add all vegetables and stir fry for 2 more minutes. Add the rest of the marinade and stir fry for a minute. Serve with brown rice or quinoa.

Pork, Green Pepper and Tomato Stir Fry

Serves 2

Ingredients - Allergies: SF, GF, DF, EF
- 1/2 pound cubed pork • 1 cup Green Peppers
- 1/2 cup sliced Tomatoes
- 1 tsp. ground black pepper
- 1 Tsp.oil

Instructions

Marinade pork in a Superfoods marinade. Stir fry drained pork in coconut oil for few minutes, add all vegetables and stir fry for 2 more minutes. Add the rest of the marinade and stir fry for a minute. Serve with brown rice or quinoa.

Pork, Red & Green Peppers, Onion & Carrots Stir Fry

Serves 2

Ingredients - Allergies: SF, GF, DF, EF
- 1/2 pound cubed pork • 1/2 cup chopped Red Peppers
- 1/2 cup chopped Green Peppers
- 1/2 cup sliced onion
- 1/2 cup sliced carrots
- 1 Tsp.oil *Instructions*

Marinade pork in a Superfoods marinade. Stir fry drained pork in coconut oil for few minutes, add all vegetables and stir fry for 2 more minutes. Add the rest of the marinade and stir fry for a minute. Serve with brown rice or quinoa.

Chicken Edamame Stir Fry

Serves 2

Ingredients - Allergies: SF, GF, DF, EF
- 1/2 pound chicken • 1 cup Edamame pre-cooked in boiling water for 3 minutes
- 1/2 cup sliced carrots
- 1 Tsp.oil

Instructions

Marinade chicken in a Superfoods marinade. Stir fry drained chicken in coconut oil for few minutes, add all vegetables and stir fry for 2 more minutes. Add the rest of the marinade and stir fry for a minute. Serve with brown rice or quinoa.

Chicken, Zucchini, Carrots and Baby Corn Stir Fry

Serves 2

Ingredients - Allergies: SF, GF, DF, EF
- 1/2 pound chicken • 1 cup Zucchini
- 1/2 cup sliced Carrots
- 1/2 cup Baby Corn
- 1 Tbsp. chopped Cilantro
- 1 Tsp.oil *Instructions*

Marinade chicken in a Superfoods marinade. Stir fry drained chicken in coconut oil for few minutes, add all vegetables and stir fry for 2 more minutes. Add the rest of the marinade and stir fry for a minute. Serve with brown rice or quinoa over bed of lettuce.

Vegan Stir Fry

Serves 2

Ingredients - Allergies: SF, GF, DF, EF, V
- 1/2 pound shiitake mushrooms • 1/2 cup Chinese Celery
- 1/2 cup sliced carrots and cucumbers
- 1 Tsp.oil *Instructions*

Marinade mushrooms in a Superfoods marinade. Stir fry drained mushrooms in coconut oil for few minutes, add all other vegetables and stir fry for 2 more minutes. Add the rest of the marinade and stir fry for a minute. Serve with brown rice or quinoa.

Eggplant, Chinese Celery & Peppers Stir Fry

Serves 2

Ingredients - Allergies: SF, GF, DF, EF, V
- 1/2 pound cubed eggplant • 1/2 cup Chinese Celery
- 1/2 cup sliced Red Peppers
- 1/4 cup sliced chili Peppers
- 1 Tsp.oil *Instructions*

Marinade eggplant in a Superfoods marinade. Stir fry drained eggplant in coconut oil for few minutes, add all vegetables and stir fry for 2 more minutes. Add the rest of the marinade and stir fry for a minute. Serve with brown rice or quinoa.

Pork Fried Brown Rice

Serves 2

Ingredients - Allergies: SF, GF, DF, EF
- 1/2 pound cubed pork • 1 cup Peppers
- 1/2 cup sliced Carrots
- 1 Tbsp. black sesame seeds
- 1 cup cooked brown rice
- 1 Tsp.oil *Instructions*

Marinade pork in a Superfoods marinade. Stir fry drained pork in coconut oil for few minutes, add all vegetables and stir fry for 2 more minutes. Add the rest of the marinade and stir fry for a minute. Stir in brown rice and black sesame seeds.

Chicken, Red Peppers, Zucchini & Cashews Stir Fry

Serves 2

Ingredients - Allergies: SF, GF, DF, EF
- 1/2 pound chicken • 1 cup Zucchini
- 1/2 cup sliced Red Peppers
- 1/2 cup sliced scallions
- 1/4 cup Cashews
- 1 Tsp.oil *Instructions*

Marinade chicken in a Superfoods marinade. Stir fry drained chicken in coconut oil for few minutes, add all vegetables and stir fry for 2 more minutes. Add the rest of the marinade and stir fry for a minute. Serve with brown rice or quinoa.

Shrimp, Asparagus, Broccoli & Carrots Stir Fry

Serves 2

Ingredients - Allergies: SF, GF, DF, EF
- 1/2 pound shrimp and calamari mix • 1/2 cup Asparagus
- 1/2 cup sliced Carrots
- 1/2 cup sliced Broccoli
- 1/2 cup sliced Chinese celery, baby corn and mushrooms
- 1 Tsp.oil *Instructions*

Marinade shrimp in a Superfoods marinade. Stir fry drained shrimp in coconut oil for few minutes, add all vegetables and stir fry for 2 more minutes. Add the rest of the marinade and stir fry for a minute. Serve with brown rice or quinoa.

Chicken, Carrots & Snow Peas Stir Fry

Serves 2
Ingredients - Allergies: SF, GF, DF, EF
- 1/2 pound chicken • 1 cup Carrots
- 1 cup Snow Peas
- 1 Tsp.oil *Instructions*

Marinade chicken in a Superfoods marinade. Stir fry drained chicken in coconut oil for few minutes, add all vegetables and stir fry for 2 more minutes. Add the rest of the marinade and stir fry for a minute. Serve with brown rice or quinoa.

Calamari, Shrimp & Bok Choy Stir Fry

Serves 2
Ingredients - Allergies: SF, GF, DF, EF
- 1 cup shrimp • 1 cup Calamari
- 1 cup sliced Bok Choy
- 1 Tsp.oil *Instructions*

Marinade calamari and shrimp in a Superfoods marinade. Stir fry drained calamari & shrimp in coconut oil for few minutes, add bok choy and stir fry for 2 more minutes. Add the rest of the marinade and stir fry for a minute. Serve with brown rice or quinoa.

Beef Liver, Chinese Celery & Mushrooms Stir Fry

Serves 2
Ingredients - Allergies: SF, GF, DF, EF
- 1/2 pound beef liver • 1 cup Chinese Celery
- 1 cup Mushrooms
- 1 Tsp.oil *Instructions*

Marinade beef liver in a Superfoods marinade. Stir fry drained beef liver in coconut oil for few minutes, add all vegetables and stir fry for 2 more minutes. Add the rest of the marinade and stir fry for a minute. Serve with brown rice or quinoa.

Chicken, Green beans & Carrot Stir Fry

Serves 2
Ingredients - Allergies: SF, GF, DF, EF
- 1/2 pound chicken • 1 cup Green Beans
- 1/2 cup chopped Carrot
- 1 Tbsp. Chia seeds
- 1 Tsp.oil *Instructions*

Marinade chicken in a Superfoods marinade. Stir fry drained chicken in coconut oil for few minutes, add all vegetables and stir fry for 2 more minutes. Add the rest of the marinade and stir fry for a minute. Serve with brown rice or quinoa.

Mixed Seafood, Spinach & Red Peppers Stir Fry

Serves 2

Ingredients - Allergies: SF, GF, DF, EF
- 1/2 pound mixed seafood • 1 cup Spinach
- 1 cup sliced Red Peppers
- 1/2 cup chopped scallions
- 1 Tsp.oil *Instructions*

Marinade seafood in a Superfoods marinade. Stir fry drained mixed seafood in coconut oil for few minutes, add red peppers and stir fry for 2 more minutes. Add the rest of the marinade and spinach and stir fry for a minute. Serve with brown rice or quinoa.

Squid, Asparagus and Red Peppers Stir Fry

Serves 2

Ingredients - Allergies: SF, GF, DF, EF
- 1/2 pound squid • 1 cup Asparagus
- 1 cup Red Peppers
- 1 Tbsp. sesame seeds
- 1 Tsp.oil *Instructions*

Marinade squid in a Superfoods marinade. Stir fry drained squid and asparagus in coconut oil for few minutes, add all other ingredients and stir fry for 2 more minutes. Add the rest of the marinade and stir fry for a minute. Serve with brown rice or quinoa.

Shrimp, Squid, Red Peppers & Green Peppers Stir Fry

Serves 2

Ingredients - Allergies: SF, GF, DF, EF
- 1/4 pound shrimp
- 1/4 pound squid • 1 cup Red peppers
- 1 cup Green peppers
- 1/4 cup Basil leaves
- 1 Tsp.oil *Instructions*

Marinade shrimp and squid in a Superfoods marinade. Stir fry drained shrimp and squid in coconut oil for few minutes, add all vegetables and stir fry for 2 more minutes. Add the rest of the marinade and stir fry for a minute. Serve with brown rice or quinoa.

Bitter Gourd, Shrimp & Peppers Stir Fry

Serves 2

Ingredients - Allergies: SF, GF, DF, EF

• 1/2 pound shrimp • 1 cup chopped Bitter Gourd pre-cooked for 2 minutes in boiling water

• 1/2 cup sliced Red peppers

• 1/4 cup Cashews

• 1 Tsp.oil *Instructions*

Marinade shrimp in a Superfoods marinade. Stir fry drained shrimp and bitter gourd in coconut oil for few minutes, add all vegetables and stir fry for 2 more minutes. Add the rest of the marinade and stir fry for a minute. Serve with brown rice or quinoa.

Pork, Mushrooms & Basil Stir Fry

Serves 2

Ingredients - Allergies: SF, GF, DF, EF

• 1/2 pound cubed pork • 1 cup sliced mushrooms

• 1/2 cup Basil leaves

• 1/2 cup sliced carrots and cucumbers

• 1 Tsp.oil *Instructions*

Marinade pork in a Superfoods marinade. Stir fry drained pork in coconut oil for few minutes, add all vegetables and stir fry for 2 more minutes. Add the rest of the marinade and stir fry for a minute. Serve with brown rice or quinoa.

Green Superfoods Stir Fry

Serves 2

Ingredients - Allergies: SF, GF, DF, EF

• 1/2 cup Kale • 1/2 cup Chinese Celery

• 1/2 cup shiitake Mushrooms

• 1/2 cup sliced Bok Choy

• 1/2 cup Asparagus

• 1 Tsp.oil *Instructions*

Marinade Asparagus and Kale in a Superfoods marinade. Stir fry drained Asparagus in coconut oil for few minutes, add all other vegetables and stir fry for 2 more minutes. Add the rest of the marinade and stir fry for a minute. Serve with brown rice or quinoa.

Pork Liver & Spinach Stir Fry

Serves 2

Ingredients - Allergies: SF, GF, DF, EF
- 1/2 pound cubed pork liver • 1 cup Spinach Celery
- 1/2 cup sliced Onions
- 1 Tsp.oil *Instructions*

Marinade pork liver in a Superfoods marinade. Stir fry drained liver in coconut oil for few minutes, add all vegetables and stir fry for 2 more minutes. Add the rest of the marinade and stir fry for a minute. Serve with brown rice or quinoa.

Squid, Shiitake Mushrooms & Basil Stir Fry

Serves 2

Ingredients - Allergies: SF, GF, DF, EF
- 1/2 pound squid • 1 cup sliced Mushrooms
- 1/2 cup Basil leaves
- 1/2 cup sliced Bok Choy
- 1/2 cup sliced carrots and red pepers
- 1 Tsp.oil *Instructions*

Marinade squid in a Superfoods marinade. Stir fry drained squid in coconut oil for few minutes, add all vegetables and stir fry for 2 more minutes. Add the rest of the marinade and stir fry for a minute. Serve with brown rice or quinoa.

Chicken, Onion & Carrot Stir Fry

Serves 2

Ingredients - Allergies: SF, GF, DF, EF
- 1/2 pound chicken • 1 cup sliced onions
- 1/2 cup sliced Bok Choy
- 1/2 cup sliced carrots and Chinese Celery
- 1 Tsp.oil *Instructions*

Marinade chicken in a Superfoods marinade. Stir fry drained chicken in coconut oil for few minutes, add all vegetables and stir fry for 2 more minutes. Add the rest of the marinade and stir fry for a minute. Serve with brown rice or quinoa.

Beef, Green beans, Broccoli & Carrot Stir Fry

Serves 2

Ingredients - Allergies: SF, GF, DF, EF
- 1/2 pound beef • 1/2 cup chopped Broccoli
- 1/2 cup chopped Green beans
- 1/2 cup sliced carrots
- 1/2 cup Baby Corn
- 1 Tsp.oil *Instructions*

Marinade beef in a Superfoods marinade. Stir fry drained beef in coconut oil for few minutes, add all vegetables and stir fry for 2 more minutes. Add the rest of the marinade and stir fry for a minute. Serve with brown rice or quinoa.

Pork, Onion & Bok Choy Stir Fry

Serves 2

Ingredients - Allergies: SF, GF, DF, EF
- 1/2 pound cubed pork • 1/2 cup sliced onions
- 1 cup sliced Bok Choy
- 1/2 cup sliced Chinese Celery
- 1 Tsp.oil *Instructions*

Marinade pork in a Superfoods marinade. Stir fry drained pork in coconut oil for few minutes, add all vegetables and stir fry for 2 more minutes. Add the rest of the marinade and stir fry for a minute. Serve with brown rice or quinoa.

Chicken, Red Peppers & Bok Choy Stir Fry

Serves 2

Ingredients - Allergies: SF, GF, DF, EF
- 1/2 pound chicken • 1/2 cup sliced onions
- 1 cup sliced Bok Choy
- 1/2 cup sliced Red Peppers
- 1 Tsp.oil *Instructions*

Marinade chicken in a Superfoods marinade. Stir fry drained chicken in coconut oil for few minutes, add all vegetables and stir fry for 2 more minutes. Add the rest of the marinade and stir fry for a minute. Serve with brown rice or quinoa.

Chicken, Eggplant & Red Peppers Stir Fry

Serves 2

Ingredients - Allergies: SF, GF, DF, EF
- 1/2 pound chicken • 1 cup sliced Eggplant
- 1/2 cup sliced Mushrooms
- 1 cup sliced Red peppers
- 1 Tsp.oil *Instructions*

Marinade chicken in a Superfoods marinade. Stir fry drained chicken in coconut oil for few minutes, add all vegetables and stir fry for 2 more minutes. Add the rest of the marinade and stir fry for a minute. Serve with brown rice or quinoa.

Pork, Cauliflower & Chinese Celery Stir Fry

Serves 2

Ingredients - Allergies: SF, GF, DF, EF
- 1/2 pound cubed pork • 1/2 cup chopped Cauliflower
- 1/2 cup sliced Broccoli
- 1/2 cup sliced Red Peppers
- 1/2 cup sliced Chinese Celery
- 1 Tsp.oil *Instructions*

Marinade pork in a Superfoods marinade. Stir fry drained pork in coconut oil for few minutes, add all vegetables and stir fry for 2 more minutes. Add the rest of the marinade and stir fry for a minute. Serve with brown rice or quinoa.

Chicken, Onion & Green & Red Peppers Stir Fry

Serves 2

Ingredients - Allergies: SF, GF, DF, EF
- 1/2 pound chicken • 1/2 cup sliced onions
- 1/2 cup sliced Green Peppers
- 1/2 cup sliced Red Peppers
- 1/2 cup Cashews
- 1 Tsp.oil *Instructions*

Marinade chicken in a Superfoods marinade. Stir fry drained chicken in coconut oil for few minutes, add all vegetables and stir fry for 2 more minutes. Add the rest of the marinade and stir fry for a minute. Serve with brown rice or quinoa.

Beef, Eggplant & Green Peppers Stir Fry

Serves 2

Ingredients - Allergies: SF, GF, DF, EF
- 1/2 pound beef • 1 cup sliced Eggplants
- 1/2 cup sliced Green peppers
- 1/2 cup sliced carrots and Chinese Celery
- 1 Tbsp. coconut oil *Instructions*

Marinade beef in a Superfoods marinade. Stir fry drained beef in coconut oil for few minutes, add all vegetables and stir fry for 2 more minutes. Add the rest of the marinade and stir fry for a minute. Serve with brown rice or quinoa.

Cauliflower & Shiitake Stir Fry

Serves 2

Ingredients - Allergies: SF, GF, DF, EF
- 2 cups Cauliflower • 1 cup sliced Shiitake mushrooms
- 1/2 cup sliced Green beans
- 1/2 cup sliced Broccoli
- 1/2 cup sliced carrot
- 1 Tbsp. coconut oil *Instructions*

Stir fry cauliflower and broccoli in coconut oil for few minutes, add carrots and green beans and stir fry for 2 more minutes. Add the mushrooms and stir fry for 3 minutes more. Serve with brown rice or quinoa.

Pork, Cabbage & Bok Choy Stir Fry

Serves 2

Ingredients - Allergies: SF, GF, DF, EF
- 1/2 pound cubed pork • 1 cup sliced Chinese cabbage
- 1/2 cup sliced bok choy
- 1/2 cup sliced red peppers
- 1 Tsp.oil *Instructions*

Marinade pork in a Superfoods marinade. Stir fry drained pork in coconut oil for few minutes, add all vegetables and stir fry for 2 more minutes. Add the rest of the marinade and stir fry for a minute. Serve with brown rice or quinoa.

Chicken & Chinese Celery Stir Fry

Serves 2

Ingredients - Allergies: SF, GF, DF, EF
- 1/2 pound chicken • 2 cups sliced Chinese Celery
- 1 Tsp.oil *Instructions*

Marinade chicken in a Superfoods marinade. Stir fry drained chicken in coconut oil for few minutes, add Chinese celery and stir fry for 2 more minutes. Add the rest of the marinade and stir fry for a minute. Serve with brown rice or quinoa.

Chicken, Broccoli & Carrots Stir Fry

Serves 2

Ingredients - Allergies: SF, GF, DF, EF
- 1/2 pound chicken • 1 cup sliced Broccoli
- 1/2 cup sliced red peppers
- 1/2 cup sliced carrots
- 1 Tsp.oil *Instructions*

Marinade chicken in a Superfoods marinade. Stir fry drained chicken in coconut oil for few minutes, add all vegetables and stir fry for 2 more minutes. Add the rest of the marinade and stir fry for a minute. Serve with brown rice or quinoa.

Chicken & Carrots Stir Fry

Serves 2

Ingredients - Allergies: SF, GF, DF, EF
- 1/2 pound chicken • 2 cup sliced Carrots
- 1/2 cup sliced onions
- 1 Tsp.oil *Instructions*

Marinade chicken in a Superfoods marinade. Stir fry drained chicken in coconut oil for few minutes, add all vegetables and stir fry for 2 more minutes. Add the rest of the marinade and stir fry for a minute. Serve with brown rice or quinoa.

Beef, Onions & Green & Red Peppers Stir Fry

Serves 2

Ingredients - Allergies: SF, GF, DF, EF
- 1/2 pound beef • 1 cup sliced Onions
- 1/2 cup sliced Green & Red peppers
- 1/2 cup sliced carrots and Celery
- 1 Tsp.oil *Instructions*

Marinade beef in a Superfoods marinade. Stir fry drained beef in coconut oil for few minutes, add all vegetables and stir fry for 2 more minutes. Add the rest of the marinade and stir fry for a minute. Serve with brown rice or quinoa.

Onions, Lentils & Tomatoes Stir Fry

Serves 2

Ingredients - Allergies: SF, GF, DF, EF
- 1/2 pound cooked lentis • 1 cup sliced Onions
- 1/2 cup sliced parsley
- 1/2 cup sliced carrots and Celery
- 1 Tsp.oil *Instructions*

Add all vegetables and stir fry for 2 more minutes. Add the lentils and stir fry for a minute. Serve with brown rice or quinoa.

Eggplant, Mushrooms & Carrots Stir Fry

Serves 2

Ingredients - Allergies: SF, GF, DF, EF
- 1/2 pound sliced Eggplant • 1 cup sliced Mushrooms
- 1/4 cup Basil leaves
- 1/2 cup sliced carrots and red peppers
- 1 Tsp.oil *Instructions*

Marinade eggplant in a Superfoods marinade. Stir fry drained eggplant in coconut oil for few minutes, add all vegetables and stir fry for 2 more minutes. Add the rest of the marinade and stir fry for a minute. Serve with brown rice or quinoa.

Chicken, Shiitake & Carrots Stir Fry

Serves 2

Ingredients - Allergies: SF, GF, DF, EF
- 1/2 pound chicken • 1 cup sliced Shiitake mushrooms
- 1/2 cup sliced Leeks
- 1/2 cup sliced carrots and Celery
- 1 Tsp.oil *Instructions*

Marinade chicken in a Superfoods marinade. Stir fry drained chicken in coconut oil for few minutes, add all vegetables and stir fry for 2 more minutes. Add the rest of the marinade and stir fry for a minute. Serve with brown rice or quinoa.

Chicken & Bok Choy Stir Fry

Serves 2

Ingredients - Allergies: SF, GF, DF, EF
- 1/2 pound chicken • 2 cups sliced Bok Choy
- 1/2 cup sliced Onions
- 1 Tbsp. oil *Instructions*

Marinade chicken in a Superfoods marinade. Stir fry drained chicken in coconut oil for few minutes, add all vegetables and stir fry for 2 more minutes. Add the rest of the marinade and stir fry for a minute. Serve with brown rice or quinoa.

Shrimp & Bok Choy Stir Fry

Serves 2

Ingredients - Allergies: SF, GF, DF, EF
- 1/2 pound shrimp • 2 cups sliced Bok Choy
- 1/2 cup sliced Green onions
- 1/2 cup sliced Chinese Celery
- 1 Tsp.oil *Instructions*

Marinade shrimp in a Superfoods marinade. Stir fry drained shrimp in coconut oil for few minutes, add all vegetables and stir fry for 2 more minutes. Add the rest of the marinade and stir fry for a minute. Serve with brown rice or quinoa.

Chicken, Green Beeans & Red Peppers Stir Fry

Serves 2

Ingredients - Allergies: SF, GF, DF, EF
- 1/2 pound chicken • 1 cup sliced Green Beans
- 1/2 cup sliced red peppers
- 1/2 cup sliced carrots and Celery
- 1 Tsp.oil *Instructions*

Marinade chicken in a Superfoods marinade. Stir fry drained chicken in coconut oil for few minutes, add all vegetables and stir fry for 2 more minutes. Add the rest of the marinade and stir fry for a minute. Serve with brown rice or quinoa.

Squid & Kimchi Stir Fry

Serves 2

Ingredients - Allergies: SF, GF, DF, EF
- 1/2 pound squid • 1 cup Kimchi
- 1/2 cup chopped green onions
- 1/4 cup chopped Cilantro
- 1 Tsp.oil *Instructions*

Marinade squid in a Superfoods marinade mixed with kimchi liquid. Stir fry drained squid in coconut oil for few minutes, add all kimchi and green onions and stir fry for 2 more minutes. Add the rest of the marinade, cilantro and stir fry for a minute. Serve with brown rice or quinoa.

Pork, Scallions & Celery Stir Fry

Serves 2

Ingredients - Allergies: SF, GF, DF, EF
- 1/2 pound cubed pork • 1 cup sliced scallions
- 1/2 cup sliced onions
- 1/2 cup sliced Celery
- 1 Tsp.oil *Instructions*

Marinade pork in a Superfoods marinade. Stir fry drained pork in coconut oil for few minutes, add all vegetables and stir fry for 2 more minutes. Add the rest of the marinade and stir fry for a minute. Serve with brown rice or quinoa.

Squid & Bitter Melon Stir Fry

Serves 2

Ingredients - Allergies: SF, GF, DF, EF
- 1/2 pound squid • 1 cup sliced Bitter Melon
- 1/2 cup sliced onions
- 1/2 cup sliced Celery
- 1 Tsp.oil *Instructions*

Marinade squid in a Superfoods marinade. Stir fry drained squid in coconut oil for few minutes, add all vegetables and stir fry for 2 more minutes. Add the rest of the marinade and stir fry for a minute. Serve with brown rice or quinoa.

Shrimp, Bok Choy & Red Peppers Stir Fry

Serves 2

Ingredients - Allergies: SF, GF, DF, EF
- 1/2 pound shrimp • 1 cup sliced Bok Choy
- 1/2 cup sliced red peppers
- 1/2 cup sliced red onions and mushrooms
- 1 Tsp.oil *Instructions*

Marinade shrimp in a Superfoods marinade. Stir fry drained shrimp in coconut oil for few minutes, add all vegetables and stir fry for 2 more minutes. Add the rest of the marinade and stir fry for a minute. Serve with brown rice or quinoa.

Pork Liver, Green Beans & Zucchini Stir Fry

Serves 2

Ingredients - Allergies: SF, GF, DF, EF
- 1/2 pound cubed pork liver • 1 cup sliced Green Beans
- 1/2 cup sliced zucchini
- 1/2 cup sliced Celery and few red chili peppers
- 1 Tsp.oil *Instructions*

Marinade liver in a Superfoods marinade. Stir fry drained liver in coconut oil for few minutes, add all vegetables and stir fry for 2 more minutes. Add the rest of the marinade and stir fry for a minute. Serve with brown rice or quinoa.

Shrimp, Edamame & Oyster Mushrooms Stir Fry

Serves 2

Ingredients - Allergies: SF, GF, DF, EF
- 1/2 pound shrimp • 1 cup shelled edamame
- 1/2 cup sliced red peppers
- 1 cup sliced oyster mushrooms
- 1 Tsp.oil *Instructions*

Marinade shrimp in a Superfoods marinade. Stir fry drained shrimp in coconut oil for few minutes, add all vegetables and stir fry for 2 more minutes. Add the rest of the marinade and stir fry for a minute. Serve with brown rice or quinoa.

Pork & Mushrooms Stir Fry

Serves 2

Ingredients - Allergies: SF, GF, DF, EF
- 1/2 pound cubed pork • 1 1/2 cup sliced mushroom
- 1 cup sliced onions
- 1 Tsp.oil *Instructions*

Marinade pork in a Superfoods marinade. Stir fry drained pork in coconut oil for few minutes, add all vegetables and stir fry for 2 more minutes. Add the rest of the marinade and stir fry for a minute. Serve with brown rice or quinoa.

Shrimp, Broccoli & Water Chestnuts Stir Fry

Serves 2

Ingredients - Allergies: SF, GF, DF, EF
- 1/2 pound shrimp • 1 cup sliced Broccoli
- 1/2 cup sliced water chestnuts
- 1/2 cup sliced Celery
- 1 Tsp.oil *Instructions*

Marinade shrimp in a Superfoods marinade. Stir fry drained shrimp in coconut oil for few minutes, add all vegetables and stir fry for 2 more minutes. Add the rest of the marinade and stir fry for a minute. Serve with brown rice or quinoa.

Mixed Seafood, Chinese Celery & Yelllow Zucchini Stir Fry

Serves 2
Ingredients - Allergies: SF, GF, DF, EF
- 1/2 pound mixed seafood • 1 cup sliced Chinese Celery
- 1/2 cup sliced bok choy
- 1/2 cup sliced onions and Celery
- 1 Tsp.oil *Instructions*

Marinade seafood in a Superfoods marinade. Stir fry drained seafood in coconut oil for few minutes, add all vegetables and stir fry for 2 more minutes. Add the rest of the marinade and stir fry for a minute. Serve with brown rice or quinoa.

Pork, Cashews & Carrots Stir Fry

Serves 2
Ingredients - Allergies: SF, GF, DF, EF
- 1/2 pound cubed pork • 1 cup sliced Green Pepper
- 1/2 cup sliced carrots
- 1/2 cup sliced onions
- 1/2 cup cashews
- 1 Tsp.oil *Instructions*

Marinade pork in a Superfoods marinade. Stir fry drained pork in coconut oil for few minutes, add all vegetables and stir fry for 2 more minutes. Add the rest of the marinade and stir fry for a minute. Serve with brown rice or quinoa.

Asparagus, Sesame Beef & Red Peppers Stir Fry

Serves 2
Ingredients - Allergies: SF, GF, DF, EF
- 1/2 pound beef • 1 cup sliced Red Pepper
- 1 cup sliced carrots
- 1/2 cup sliced onions
- 1/2 sesame seeds
- 1 Tsp.oil *Instructions*

Marinade beef in a Superfoods marinade. Roll drained beef in sesame seeds and stir fry in coconut oil for few minutes with asparagus. Add other vegetables and stir fry for 4 more minutes. Add the rest of the marinade and stir fry for a minute. Serve with brown rice or quinoa.

Baby Corn, Mushrooms & Asparagus Stir Fry

Serves 2

Ingredients - Allergies: SF, GF, DF, EF
- 1 cup mushrooms • 1/2 cup Baby corn
- 1/2 cup sliced green beans
- 1/2 cup sliced yellow peppers
- 1/2 cup asparagus
- 1 Tsp.oil *Instructions*

Stir fry asparagus, green beans and baby corn in coconut oil for few minutes, add peppers and mushrooms and stir fry for 2 more minutes. Add the superfoods marinade and stir fry for a minute. Serve with brown rice or quinoa.

Chinese Broccoli, Chicken & Cherry Tomatoes Stir Fry

Serves 2

Ingredients - Allergies: SF, GF, DF, EF
- 1/2 pound chicken • 1 cup sliced Chinese broccoli
- 1 cup halved cherry tomatoes
- 1/4 cup sliced onions
- 1/2 cup cashews
- 1 Tsp.oil *Instructions*

Marinade chicken in a Superfoods marinade. Stir fry drained chicken in coconut oil for few minutes, add all vegetables and stir fry for 2 more minutes. Add the rest of the marinade and stir fry for a minute. Serve with brown rice or quinoa.

Baby Squid, Sprouts & Spring Onions Stir Fry

Serves 2

Ingredients - Allergies: SF, GF, DF, EF
- 1/2 pound baby squid • 1 cup sprouts
- 1/2 cup sliced spring onions
- 1/2 cup sliced red peppers
- 1/4 cup chili sauce (mix chili flakes with oil and salt)
- 1 tsp. minced garlic and ginger each
- 1 Tsp.oil *Instructions*

Marinade baby squid in a chili sauce, garlic and ginger. Stir fry drained squid in coconut oil for few minutes, add all vegetables and stir fry for 2 more minutes. Add the rest of the marinade (if any) and stir fry for a minute. Serve with brown rice or quinoa.

Chinese Eggplant, Lotus Root & Chicken Stir Fry

Serves 2

Ingredients - Allergies: SF, GF, DF, EF

- 1/2 pound chicken • 1 cup sliced Chinese eggplant
- 1/2 cup sliced carrots
- 1/2 cup sliced onions
- 1/2 cup sliced lotus root
- 1 Tsp.oil *Instructions*

Marinade chicken and eggplant in a Superfoods marinade. Stir fry drained chicken and eggplant in coconut oil for few minutes, add all vegetables and stir fry for 2 more minutes. Add the rest of the marinade and stir fry for a minute. Serve with brown rice or quinoa.

Green Beans, Chicken Chili Sauce & Onions Stir Fry

Serves 2

Ingredients - Allergies: SF, GF, DF, EF

- 1/2 pound chicken • 1 cup sliced Green Beans
- 1/2 cup sliced onions
- 1/4 cup chili sauce (mix chili flakes with oil and salt)
- 1 tsp. minced garlic and ginger each
- 1 Tsp.oil *Instructions*

Marinade chicken in a chili sauce, ginger and garlic. Stir fry drained chicken in coconut oil for few minutes, add all vegetables and stir fry for 2 more minutes. Add the rest of the marinade and stir fry for a minute. Serve with brown rice or quinoa.

Asparagus, Shrimp & Mushrooms Stir Fry

Serves 2

Ingredients - Allergies: SF, GF, DF, EF

- 1/2 pound shrimp • 1 cup sliced Asparagus
- 1 cup sliced mushrooms
- 1 Tsp.oil *Instructions*

Marinade shrimp in a Superfoods marinade. Stir fry drained shrimp in coconut oil for few minutes, add all vegetables and stir fry for 2 more minutes. Add the rest of the marinade and stir fry for a minute. Serve with brown rice or quinoa.

Edamame, Asparagus, Pork & Snow Peas Stir Fry

Serves 2
Ingredients - Allergies: SF, GF, DF, EF
- 1/2 pound cubed pork • 1 cup sliced Asparagus
- 1/2 cup snow peas
- 1/2 cup sliced onions
- 1/2 cup edamame
- 1 Tsp.oil *Instructions*

Marinade pork in a Superfoods marinade. Stir fry drained pork in coconut oil for few minutes, add all vegetables and stir fry for 2 more minutes. Add the rest of the marinade and stir fry for a minute. Serve with brown rice or quinoa.

Snow Peas, Shrimp & Bok Choy Stir Fry

Serves 2
Ingredients - Allergies: SF, GF, DF, EF
- 1/2 pound shrimp • 1 cup sliced Green Peas
- 1 cup sliced bok choy
- 1/2 cup sliced onions
- 1 Tsp.oil *Instructions*

Marinade shrimp in a Superfoods marinade. Stir fry drained shrimp in coconut oil for few minutes, add all vegetables and stir fry for 2 more minutes. Add the rest of the marinade and stir fry for a minute. Serve with brown rice or quinoa.

Sprouts, Shrimp & Julienned Carrots Stir Fry

Serves 2
Ingredients - Allergies: SF, GF, DF, EF
- 1/2 pound shrimp • 1 cup Sprouts
- 1/2 cup julienned carrots
- 1/2 cup sliced onions
- 1 Tsp.oil *Instructions*

Marinade shrimp in a Superfoods marinade. Stir fry drained shrimp in coconut oil for few minutes, add all vegetables and stir fry for 2 more minutes. Add the rest of the marinade and stir fry for a minute. Serve with brown rice or quinoa.

Water Chestnut, Chicken & Broccoli Stir Fry

Serves 2

Ingredients - Allergies: SF, GF, DF, EF
- 1/2 pound cubed pork • 1 cup sliced Broccoli
- 1/2 cup sliced celery
- 1/2 cup sliced onions
- 1 cup sliced water chestnuts
- 1 Tsp.oil *Instructions*

Marinade pork in a Superfoods marinade. Stir fry drained pork in coconut oil for few minutes, add all vegetables and stir fry for 2 more minutes. Add the rest of the marinade and stir fry for a minute. Serve with brown rice or quinoa.

Asparagus, Red Peppers & Pork Stir Fry

Serves 2

Ingredients - Allergies: SF, GF, DF, EF
- 1/2 pound cubed pork • 1 cup sliced Asparagus
- 1/2 cup sliced celery
- 1/2 cup sliced onions
- 1 cup sliced Red Peppers
- 1 Tsp.oil *Instructions*

Marinade pork in a Superfoods marinade. Stir fry drained pork in coconut oil for few minutes, add all vegetables and stir fry for 2 more minutes. Add the rest of the marinade and stir fry for a minute. Serve with brown rice or quinoa.

Baby Corn, Shrimp, Sprouts & Broccoli Stir Fry

Serves 2

Ingredients - Allergies: SF, GF, DF, EF
- 1/2 pound shrimp • 1 cup sliced Broccoli
- 1/2 cup julienned carrots
- 1/2 cup sprouts
- 1 cup baby corn
- 1 Tsp.oil *Instructions*

Marinade shrimp in a Superfoods marinade. Stir fry drained shrimp in coconut oil for few minutes, add all vegetables and stir fry for 2 more minutes. Add the rest of the marinade and stir fry for a minute. Serve with brown rice or quinoa.

Beef Broth, Asparagus & Onions Stir Fry

Serves 2

Ingredients - Allergies: SF, GF, DF, EF

- 1/2 pound cubed beef • 2 cups asparagus
- 1/2 cup sliced celery
- 1/2 cup sliced onion
- 1 Tsp.oil *Instructions*

Marinade beef in a Superfoods marinade. Stir fry drained beef in coconut oil for few minutes, add all vegetables and stir fry for 2 more minutes. Add the rest of the marinade and stir fry for a minute. Serve with brown rice or quinoa.

Green Beans, Cashews & Pork Stir Fry

Serves 2

Ingredients - Allergies: SF, GF, DF, EF

- 1/2 pound cubed pork • 1 cup sliced green beans
- 1/2 cup sliced celery
- 1/2 cup sliced onions
- 1/2 cup cashews
- 1 Tsp.oil *Instructions*

Marinade pork in a Superfoods marinade. Stir fry drained pork in coconut oil for few minutes, add all vegetables and stir fry for 2 more minutes. Add the rest of the marinade and stir fry for a minute. Serve with brown rice or quinoa.

Pineapple, Red Pepers, Onions & Beef Stir Fry

Serves 2

Ingredients - Allergies: SF, GF, DF, EF

- 1/2 pound cubed beef • 1 cup sliced pineapple
- 1/2 cup sliced Red peppers
- 1/2 cup sliced onions
- 1/2 cup sliced Green peppers
- 1 Tsp.oil *Instructions*

Marinade beef in a Superfoods marinade. Stir fry drained beef in coconut oil for few minutes, add all vegetables and stir fry for 2 more minutes. Add the rest of the marinade and stir fry for a minute. Serve with brown rice or quinoa.

Carrot, Chicken, Onions & Broccoli Stir Fry

Serves 2

Ingredients - Allergies: SF, GF, DF, EF
- 1/2 pound cubed chicken • 1 cup sliced Broccoli
- 1/2 cup sliced celery
- 1/2 cup sliced green onions
- 1/2 cup sliced carrots
- 1 Tsp.oil *Instructions*

Marinade chicken in a Superfoods marinade. Stir fry drained chicken in coconut oil for few minutes, add all vegetables and stir fry for 2 more minutes. Add the rest of the marinade and stir fry for a minute. Serve with brown rice or quinoa.

Eggplant, Green Peppers & Minced Pork Stir Fry

Serves 2

Ingredients - Allergies: SF, GF, DF, EF
- 1/2 pound minced pork • 2 cups sliced eggplant
- 1/2 cup sliced celery
- 1/2 cup sliced onions
- 1/2 cup sliced carrot
- 1 Tsp.oil *Instructions*

Marinade pork in a Superfoods marinade. Stir fry drained pork in coconut oil for few minutes, add all vegetables and stir fry for 2 more minutes. Add the rest of the marinade and stir fry for a minute. Serve with brown rice or quinoa.

Chives, Carrot & Pork Stir Fry

Serves 2

Ingredients - Allergies: SF, GF, DF, EF
- 1/2 pound cubed pork • 1 + 1/2 cup chives
- 1/2 cup sliced celery
- 1/2 cup sliced onions
- 1/2 cup sliced carrot
- 1 Tsp.oil *Instructions*

Marinade pork in a Superfoods marinade. Stir fry drained pork in coconut oil for few minutes, add all vegetables and stir fry for 2 more minutes. Add the rest of the marinade and stir fry for a minute. Serve with brown rice or quinoa.

Green Onions, Ground Cashews & Pork Stir Fry

Serves 2
Ingredients - Allergies: SF, GF, DF, EF
- 1/2 pound cubed pork • 1 cup sliced Green onions
- 1/2 cup sliced celery
- 1/2 cup sliced Green Peppers
- 1/2 cup ground cashews
- 1 Tsp.oil *Instructions*

Marinade pork in a Superfoods marinade. Stir fry drained pork in coconut oil for few minutes, add all vegetables and stir fry for 2 more minutes. Add the rest of the marinade and stir fry for a minute. Serve with brown rice or quinoa.

Asparagus, Shrimp & Sprouts Stir Fry

Serves 2
Ingredients - Allergies: SF, GF, DF, EF
- 1/2 pound shrimp • 2 cups sliced Asparagus
- 1/2 cup sliced celery
- 1/2 cup sliced onions
- 1 Tbsp. coconut oil

Instructions

Marinade shrimp in a Superfoods marinade. Stir fry drained shrimp in coconut oil for few minutes, add all vegetables and stir fry for 2 more minutes. Add the rest of the marinade and stir fry for a minute. Serve with brown rice or quinoa.

Baby Corn, Snow Peas & Chicken Stir Fry

Serves 2
Ingredients - Allergies: SF, GF, DF, EF
- 1/2 pound chicken • 1 cup baby corn
- 1/2 cup snow peas
- 1/2 cup julienned carrot
- 1/2 cup sliced mushrooms
- 1/2 cup sliced red peppers
- 1 Tbsp. coconut oil

Instructions

Marinade shrimp in a Superfoods marinade. Stir fry drained chicken in coconut oil for few minutes, add all vegetables and stir fry for 2 more minutes. Add the rest of the marinade and stir fry for a minute. Serve with brown rice or quinoa.

Bamboo Shoots & Chinese Celery Stir Fry

Serves 2

Ingredients - Allergies: SF, GF, DF, EF
- 3 cups sliced bamboo shoots • 2 cups sliced Chinese celery
- 1/2 cup sliced onions
- 1 Tbsp. coconut oil

Instructions

Stir fry bamboo shoots in coconut oil for few minutes, add Chinese celery and onions and stir fry for 2 more minutes. Add the superfoods marinade and stir fry for a minute. Serve with brown rice or quinoa.

Carrot, Sesame & Spicy Beef Stir Fry

Serves 2

Ingredients - Allergies: SF, GF, DF, EF
- 1/2 pound beef • 2 cups sliced carrots
- 1/2 cup sesame seeds
- 1/2 cup sliced onions
- 1 Tbsp. coconut oil

Instructions

Marinade shrimp in a Superfoods marinade (add 1 Tbsp. ground cumin). Stir fry beef in coconut oil for few minutes, add all vegetables and stir fry for 2 more minutes. Add the rest of the marinade and stir fry for a minute. Sprinkle with sesame seeds and serve with brown rice or quinoa.

Green Pepper, Onion & BlackPeper Beef Stir Fry

Serves 2

Ingredients - Allergies: SF, GF, DF, EF
- 1/2 pound beef stripes • 1 cup sliced green pepper
- 1/2 cup sliced celery
- 1/2 cup sliced onions
- 1 Tbsp. coconut oil
- 1 Tsp. black pepper

Instructions

Marinade beef in a Superfoods marinade (add 1Tbsp. black pepper). Stir fry drained beef in coconut oil for few minutes, add all vegetables and stir fry for 2 more minutes. Add the rest of the marinade and stir fry for a minute. Serve with brown rice or quinoa.

String Beans, Onion & Beef Stir Fry

Serves 2
Ingredients - Allergies: SF, GF, DF, EF
- 1/2 pound beef • 2 cups sliced string onion
- 1/2 cup sliced onions
- 1 red chili pepper
- 1 Tbsp. coconut oil
Instructions
Marinade shrimp in a Superfoods marinade. Stir fry drained shrimp in coconut oil for few minutes, add all vegetables and stir fry for 2 more minutes. Add the rest of the marinade and stir fry for a minute. Serve with brown rice or quinoa.

Cumin Beef & Spinach Stir Fry

Serves 2
Ingredients - Allergies: SF, GF, DF, EF
- 1/2 pound beef • 1 cup sliced Spinach
- 1 cup sliced Chinese celery
- 1/2 cup sliced onions
- 1 Tbsp. coconut oil
- 2 Tsp. ground cumin
Instructions
Marinade beef in a Superfoods marinade (add ground cumin). Stir fry drained beef in coconut oil for few minutes, add onions and Chinese celery and stir fry for 2 more minutes. Add the rest of the marinade and spinach and stir fry for a minute. Serve with brown rice or quinoa.

Bitter Gourd & Minced Meat Stir Fry

Serves 2
Ingredients - Allergies: SF, GF, DF, EF
- 1/2 pound minced beef • 2 cups sliced bitter gourd
- 1/2 cup sprouts
- 1/2 cup sliced onions
- 1 Tbsp. coconut oil
Instructions
Marinade minced beef in a Superfoods marinade. Stir fry drained minced beef in coconut oil for few minutes, add all vegetables and stir fry for 2 more minutes. Add the rest of the marinade and stir fry for a minute. Serve with brown rice or quinoa.

Chicken, Mushrooms & Asparagus Stir Fry

Serves 2

Ingredients - Allergies: SF, GF, DF, EF
- 1/2 pound chicken breast meat • 1 cups sliced Asparagus
- 1/2 cup sliced carrot
- 1/2 cup sliced mushrooms
- 1 Tbsp. coconut oil

Instructions

Marinade chicken in a Superfoods marinade. Stir fry drained chicken in coconut oil for few minutes, add all vegetables and stir fry for 2 more minutes. Add the rest of the marinade and stir fry for a minute. Serve with brown rice or quinoa.

Snow Peas, Chicken & Asparagus Stir Fry

Serves 2

Ingredients - Allergies: SF, GF, DF, EF
- 1/2 pound chicken • 2 cups sliced snow peas
- 1/2 cup sliced asparagus
- 1/2 cup julienned carrots
- 1 Tbsp. coconut oil

Instructions

Marinade chicken in a Superfoods marinade. Stir fry drained chicken in coconut oil for few minutes, add all vegetables and stir fry for 2 more minutes. Add the rest of the marinade and stir fry for a minute. Serve with brown rice or quinoa.

Fish, Sprouts, Chinese Celery & Dill Stir Fry

Serves 2

Ingredients - Allergies: SF, GF, DF, EF
- 1/2 pound fish of your choice • 2 cups sprouts
- 2 cup sliced Chinese celery
- 1/2 cup sliced dill
- 1 Tbsp. coconut oil

Instructions

Marinade fish in a Superfoods marinade. Stir fry drained fish in coconut oil for few minutes, add all vegetables and stir fry for 2 more minutes. Add the rest of the marinade and stir fry for a minute. Serve with brown rice or quinoa.

Beef & Snow Peas Stir Fry

Serves 2

Ingredients - Allergies: SF, GF, DF, EF
- 1/2 pound beef • 2 cups sliced Snow Peas
- 1/2 of the small onion, sliced
- 1 Tbsp. coconut oil
- 1 Tsp. red pepper flakes

Instructions

Marinade beef in a Superfoods marinade (add red pepper flakes). Stir fry drained beef in coconut oil for few minutes, add onions and Snow Peas and stir fry for 2 more minutes. Add the rest of the marinade and stir fry for a minute. Serve with brown rice or quinoa.

Beef & Yellow Peppers Stir Fry

Serves 2

Ingredients - Allergies: SF, GF, DF, EF
- 1/2 pound beef • 2 sliced Yellow Peppers
- 1 sliced Red or Orange pepper
- 1/2 cup sliced onions
- 1 Tbsp. coconut oil
- 1/2 cup broccoli florets
- 1/2 cup mushrooms
- 1/2 cup sliced zucchini or celery or both

Instructions

Marinade beef in a Superfoods marinade. Stir fry drained beef in coconut oil for few minutes, add all veggies and stir fry for 2 more minutes. Add the rest of the marinade and stir fry for a minute. Serve with brown rice or quinoa.

Bok Choy & Seaweed Stir Fry

Serves 2

Ingredients - Allergies: SF, GF, DF, EF
- 2 cups sliced Bok Choy
- 1/2 cup dried mixed seaweed
- 1/2 cup julienned carrots
- 2 tbsp. bonito flakes
- 1 Tbsp. coconut oil

Instructions

Put the dried seaweed in lots of water and soak for 10-15 minutes. At the same time marinade sliced bok choy in Superfoods marinade for 15 minutes. Stir fry drained bok choy in coconut oil for 1 minute, add carrots, squeezed out seaweed and the rest of the marinade and stir fry for 1 more minute. Top with bonito flakes. Serve with brown rice or quinoa.

Chicken & Bok Choy Stir Fry

Serves 2

Ingredients - Allergies: SF, GF, DF, EF
- 1/2 pound chicken • 2 cups sliced Bok Choy
- 1/4 cup sliced Chinese celery
- 1/2 cup sliced onions
- 1 Tbsp. coconut oil

Instructions

Marinade chicken in a Superfoods marinade. Stir fry drained chicken in coconut oil for few minutes, add onions and Chinese celery and stir fry for 2 more minutes. Add the rest of the marinade and bok choy and stir fry for a minute. Serve with brown rice or quinoa.

Chicken, Bok Choy, Snow Peas & Peanuts Stir Fry

Serves 2

Ingredients - Allergies: SF, GF, DF, EF
- 1/2 pound chicken • 1 cup sliced Bok choy
- 1 cup Snow Peas
- 1/2 cup sliced onions
- 1 Tbsp. coconut oil
- 2 Tbsp. peanuts

Instructions

Marinade chicken in a Superfoods marinade. Stir fry drained chicken and peanuts in coconut oil for few minutes, add onions, snow peas and bok choy and stir fry for 2 more minutes. Add the rest of the marinade and stir fry for a minute. Serve with brown rice or quinoa.

Mongolian Stir Fry

Serves 2

Ingredients - Allergies: SF, GF, DF, EF
- 1/2 pound beef • 1 cup sliced zucchini
- 1 cup sliced carrots
- 1/2 cup sliced onions
- 1/2 cup sliced green peppers
- 1 Tbsp. coconut oil
- 2 Tsp. ground cumin

Instructions

Marinade beef, carrots and zucchini in a Superfoods marinade (add ground cumin). Stir fry drained beef and veggies in coconut oil for few minutes, add onions and green peppers and stir fry for 2 more minutes. Add the rest of the marinade and stir fry for a minute. Serve with brown rice or quinoa.

Mushrooms, Snow Peas & Bok Choy Stir Fry

Serves 2

Ingredients - Allergies: SF, GF, DF, EF
- 1/2 pound mushrooms • 1 cup Snow Peas
- 1 cup sliced Bok Choy
- 1/2 cup sliced onions
- 1 Tbsp. coconut oil

Instructions

Marinade mushrooms in a Superfoods marinade. Stir fry drained mushrooms in coconut oil for few minutes, add onions and Snow Peas and stir fry for 2 more minutes. Add the rest of the marinade and bok choy and stir fry for a minute. Serve with brown rice or quinoa.

Pork, Red Peppers, Carrots, Celery & Basil Stir Fry

Serves 2

Ingredients - Allergies: SF, GF, DF, EF
- 1/2 pound cubed pork • 1 cup sliced Red Peppers
- 1/2 cup sliced celery
- 1/2 cup sliced carrots
- 1 Tbsp. coconut oil
- 2 Tbsp. sliced Basil leaves

Instructions

Marinade pork in a Superfoods marinade. Stir fry drained pork in coconut oil for few minutes, add carrots and celery and stir fry for 2 more minutes. Add the rest of the marinade and basil leaves and stir fry for a minute. Serve with brown rice or quinoa.

Pork, Zucchini & Onions Stir Fry

Serves 2

Ingredients - Allergies: SF, GF, DF, EF
- 1/2 pound pork • 1 cup sliced Zucchini
- 1 cup sliced onions
- 1 Tbsp. coconut oil

Instructions

Marinade pork in a Superfoods marinade. Stir fry drained pork in coconut oil for few minutes, add zucchini and onions and stir fry for 2 more minutes. Add the rest of the marinade and stir fry for a minute. Serve with brown rice or quinoa.

Snow Peas, Shrimp, Mushrooms & Bok Choy Stir Fry

Serves 2

Ingredients - Allergies: SF, GF, DF, EF

- 1/2 pound shrimp • 1 cup sliced Snow peas
- 1 cup sliced Chinese celery
- 1/2 cup sliced mushrooms
- 1 Tbsp. coconut oil

Instructions

Marinade shrimp in a Superfoods marinade. Stir fry drained shrimp in coconut oil for few minutes, add snow peas and Chinese celery and stir fry for 2 more minutes. Add the rest of the marinade and mushrooms and stir fry for a minute. Serve with brown rice or quinoa.

Eggplant, Red Peppers & Carrots Stir Fry

Serves 2

Ingredients - Allergies: SF, GF, DF, EF

- 1/2 pound Red Peppers • 1 + 1/2 cup sliced Eggplant
- 1 cup sliced Carrots
- 1/2 cup sliced onions
- 1 Tbsp. coconut oil

Instructions

Marinade eggplant in a Superfoods marinade. Stir fry drained eggplant and carrots in coconut oil for 5 minutes, add red peppers and onions, stir fry for 2 more minutes. Add the rest of the marinade and stir fry for a minute. Serve with brown rice or quinoa.

Eggplant, Shiitake & Bamboo Shoots Stir Fry

Serves 2

Ingredients - Allergies: SF, GF, DF, EF

- 1/2 pound sliced shiitake mushrooms • 1 cup sliced eggplant
- 1 cup sliced Green peppers
- 1/2 cup sliced carrots
- 1/2 cup sliced onions
- 1/2 cup sliced bamboo shoots
- 1 Tbsp. coconut oil

Instructions

Marinade shiitake, bamboo shoots and eggplant in a Superfoods marinade. Stir fry drained eggplant and bamboo shoots in coconut oil for 5 minutes, add carrots and onions and stir fry for 2 more minutes. Add the rest of the marinade with shiitake and stir fry for a minute. Serve with brown rice or quinoa.

Korean Squid Stir Fry

Serves 2

Ingredients - Allergies: SF, GF, DF, EF
- 1 pound Squid stripes • 1 cup sliced carrots
- 1/2 cup Korean Spicy marinade
- 1/2 cup sliced onions
- 1 Tbsp. coconut oil

Instructions

Marinade squid stripes in a Korean spicy marinade. Stir fry drained squid in coconut oil for few minutes, add carrots and onions and stir fry for 2 more minutes. Add the rest of the marinade and stir fry for a minute. Serve with brown rice or quinoa.

Okra, Sprouts & Onions Choy Stir Fry

Serves 2

Ingredients - Allergies: SF, GF, DF, EF
- 1 + 1/2 pound sliced okra • 1 cup sprouts
- 1/2 cup sliced onions
- 1 Tbsp. coconut oil

Instructions

Marinade okra in a Superfoods marinade. Stir fry drained okra in coconut oil for few minutes, add onions and stir fry for 2 more minutes. Add the rest of the marinade and sprouts and stir fry for a minute. Serve with brown rice or quinoa.

Okra, Asparagus, Chicken & Onions Stir Fry

Serves 2

Ingredients - Allergies: SF, GF, DF, EF
- 1/2 pound chicken • 1 cup sliced okra
- 1 cup sliced asparagus
- 1/2 cup sliced onions
- 1 Tbsp. coconut oil

Instructions

Marinade chicken in a Korean Spicy marinade. Stir fry drained chicken in coconut oil for few minutes, add okra and asparagus and stir fry for 2 more minutes. Add the rest of the marinade and onions and stir fry for a minute. Serve with brown rice or quinoa.

Okra, Ground Beef, Red Peppers & Cilantro Stir Fry

Serves 2

Ingredients - Allergies: SF, GF, DF, EF

- 1/2 pound ground beef • 1 cup sliced okra
- 1 cup sliced red peppers
- 1/2 cup sliced onions
- 1/4 cup sliced cilantro
- 1 Tbsp. coconut oil

Instructions

Marinade okra in a Superfoods marinade. Stir fry drained okra and ground beef in coconut oil for few minutes, add red peppers and onions and stir fry for 2 more minutes. Add the rest of the marinade and half of cilantro and stir fry for a minute. Decorate with the rest of cilantro. Serve with brown rice or quinoa.

Pork, Broccoli, Baby Carrots & Mushrooms Stir Fry

Serves 2

Ingredients - Allergies: SF, GF, DF, EF

- 1/2 pound cubed pork • 1 cup sliced Broccoli
- 1 cup halved lengthwise baby carrots
- 1/2 cup sliced mushrooms
- 1 Tbsp. coconut oil

Instructions

Marinade pork in a Superfoods marinade. Stir fry drained pork in coconut oil for few minutes, add broccoli and baby carrots and stir fry for 2 more minutes. Add the rest of the marinade and mushrooms and stir fry for a minute. Serve with brown rice or quinoa.

Pork, Red Peppers, Broccoli & Carrots Stir Fry

Serves 2

Ingredients - Allergies: SF, GF, DF, EF

- 1/2 pound pork • 1 cup sliced Red Peppers
- 1 cup sliced Broccoli
- 1/2 cup sliced carrots
- 1 Tbsp. coconut oil

Instructions

Marinade pork in a Superfoods marinade. Stir fry drained pork in coconut oil for few minutes, add broccoli and carrots and stir fry for 2 more minutes. Add the rest of the marinade and red peppers and stir fry for a minute. Serve with brown rice or quinoa.

Green Peas, Pork, Onions & Cilntro Stir Fry

Serves 2

Ingredients - Allergies: SF, GF, DF, EF
- 1/2 pound pork • 1 cup Green peas
- 1 cup sliced onions
- 1/4 cup cilantro
- 1 Tbsp. coconut oil

Instructions

Marinade pork in a Superfoods marinade. Stir fry drained pork and green peas in coconut oil for few minutes, add onions and stir fry for 2 more minutes. Add the rest of the marinade and stir fry for a minute. Serve with brown rice or quinoa.

Bitter Gourd, Shrimp & Squid Stir Fry

Serves 2

Ingredients - Allergies: SF, GF, DF, EF
- 1/2 pound squid slices • 1/2 pound shrimp
- 1 cup sliced bitter gourd
- 1/2 cup sliced onions
- 1 Tbsp. coconut oil

Instructions

Marinade shrimp and squid in a Superfoods marinade. Stir fry drained shrimp and squid in coconut oil for few minutes, add bitter gourd and stir fry for 2 more minutes. Add the rest of the marinade and onions and stir fry for a minute. Serve with brown rice or quinoa.

Baby Carrots & Shrimp Stir Fry

Serves 2

Ingredients - Allergies: SF, GF, DF, EF
- 1/2 pound shrimp • 1 cup baby carrots
- 1/2 cup sliced Broccoli
- 1/2 cup sliced mushrooms
- 1 Tbsp. coconut oil

Instructions

Marinade pork in a Superfoods marinade. Stir fry drained shrimp in coconut oil for few minutes, add broccoli and carrots and stir fry for 2 more minutes. Add the rest of the marinade and mushrooms and stir fry for a minute. Serve with brown rice or quinoa.

Beef, Onions & Chili Stir Fry

Serves 2
Ingredients - Allergies: SF, GF, DF, EF
- 1/2 pound beef • 1 cup sliced onions
- 1/2 cup sliced celery
- 1 Tbsp. coconut oil
- 1 Tsp. chili sauce (to taste)

Instructions
Marinade pork in a Superfoods marinade with chili sauce added. Stir fry drained beef in coconut oil for few minutes, add onions and celery and stir fry for 2 more minutes. Add the rest of the marinade and red peppers and stir fry for a minute. Serve with brown rice or quinoa.

Black Pepper Beef & Green Peppers Stir Fry

Serves 2
Ingredients - Allergies: SF, GF, DF, EF
- 1/2 pound beef • 1 cup sliced Green Peppers
- 1 cup sliced Onion
- 1/2 cup sliced celery
- 1 Tbsp. coconut oil

Instructions
Marinade beef in a Superfoods marinade. Stir fry drained beef in coconut oil for few minutes, add celery and onions and stir fry for 2 more minutes. Add the rest of the marinade and green peppers and stir fry for a minute. Serve with brown rice or quinoa.

Lamb, Mushrooms & Broccoli Stir Fry

Serves 2
Ingredients - Allergies: SF, GF, DF, EF
- 1/2 pound lamb • 1 cup sliced Mushrooms
- 1 cup sliced Broccoli
- 1/2 cup sliced onions
- 1 Tbsp. coconut oil

Instructions
Marinade lamb in a Superfoods marinade. Stir fry drained lamb in coconut oil for few minutes, add broccoli and onions and stir fry for 2 more minutes. Add the rest of the marinade and mushrooms and stir fry for a minute. Serve with brown rice or quinoa.

Pork, Carrots & Spinach Stir Fry

Serves 2

Ingredients - Allergies: SF, GF, DF, EF
- 1/2 pound pork • 1 cup spinach
- 1 cup sliced carrots
- 1 Tbsp. coconut oil

Instructions

Marinade pork in a Superfoods marinade. Stir fry drained pork in coconut oil for few minutes, add carrots and stir fry for 2 more minutes. Add the rest of the marinade and spinach and stir fry for a minute. Serve with brown rice or quinoa.

Pork, Bok Choy & GreenPeppers Stir Fry

Serves 2

Ingredients - Allergies: SF, GF, DF, EF
- 1/2 pound pork • 1 cup sliced Green Peppers
- 1 cup sliced Bok Choy
- 1/2 cup sliced green onions
- 1 Tbsp. coconut oil

Instructions

Marinade pork in a Superfoods marinade. Stir fry drained pork in coconut oil for few minutes, add white parts of bok choy and green onions and stir fry for 2 more minutes. Add the rest of the marinade and green peppers and the rest of bok choy and stir fry for a minute. Serve with brown rice or quinoa.

Pork, Green Onions & Red Peppers Stir Fry

Serves 2

Ingredients - Allergies: SF, GF, DF, EF
- 1/2 pound pork • 1 cup sliced Red Peppers
- 1 cup sliced green onions
- 1/2 cup sliced carrots
- 1 Tbsp. coconut oil

Instructions

Marinade pork in a Superfoods marinade. Stir fry drained pork in coconut oil for few minutes, add green onions and carrots and stir fry for 2 more minutes. Add the rest of the marinade and red peppers and stir fry for a minute. Serve with brown rice or quinoa.

Squid, Chinese Cabbage, Green Onions, Zucchini & Chili Pepper Paste Stir Fry

Serves 2

Ingredients - Allergies: SF, GF, DF, EF
- 1/2 pound squid • 1 cup sliced Chinese cabbage
- 1 cup sliced Zucchini
- 1/2 cup sliced green onions
- 1 Tsp. chili paste (to taste)
- 1 Tbsp. coconut oil

Instructions

Marinade squid in a Superfoods marinade with chili sauce. Stir fry drained squid in coconut oil for few minutes, add green onions and zucchini and stir fry for 2 more minutes. Add the rest of the marinade and Chinese cabbage and stir fry for a minute. Serve with brown rice or quinoa.

Water Chectnut, Shrimp & Broccoli Stir Fry

Serves 2

Ingredients - Allergies: SF, GF, DF, EF
- 1/2 pound shrimp • 1 cup sliced Broccoli
- 1/2 cup sliced water chestnuts
- 1 Tbsp. coconut oil

Instructions

Marinade shrimp in a Superfoods marinade. Stir fry drained shrimp in coconut oil for few minutes, add broccoli and water chestnuts and stir fry for 2 more minutes. Add the rest of the marinade and stir fry for a minute. Serve with brown rice or quinoa.

Zucchini, Peppers, Carrots, Mushrooms & Green Beans Stir Fry

Serves 2

Ingredients - Allergies: SF, GF, DF, EF
- 1/2 cup sliced mushrooms • 1/2 cup sliced Red Peppers
- 1/2 cup sliced Zucchini
- 1/2 cup sliced carrots
- 1/2 cup sliced green beans
- 1/2 cup sliced green onions
- 1 Tbsp. coconut oil

Instructions

Marinade zucchini in a Superfoods marinade. Stir fry drained zucchini in coconut oil for few minutes, add all other veggies and stir fry for 4 more minutes. Add the rest of the marinade and stir fry for a minute. Serve with brown rice or quinoa.

Beef, Shitake, Brocoli & Red PeppersStir Fry

Serves 2

Ingredients - Allergies: SF, GF, DF, EF
- 1/2 pound beef • 1/2 cup sliced Broccoli
- 1/2 cup halved shiitake
- 1/2 cup sliced red peppers
- 1 Tbsp. coconut oil

Instructions

Marinade shrimp in a Superfoods marinade. Stir fry drained beef in coconut oil for few minutes, add all veggies and stir fry for 2 more minutes. Add the rest of the marinade and stir fry for a minute. Serve with brown rice or quinoa.

Bok Choy, Celery & Onions Stir Fry

Serves 2

Ingredients - Allergies: SF, GF, DF, EF
- 1/2 pound Bok Choy, sliced • 1 cup sliced Celery
- 1/2 cup chopped onions
- 1 Tbsp. coconut oil

Instructions

Marinade white part of bok choy in a Superfoods marinade. Stir fry drained bok choy in coconut oil for 2 minutes, add celery and onions and stir fry for 2 more minutes. Add sliced green parts of bok choy and the rest of the marinade and stir fry for a minute. Serve with brown rice or quinoa.

Chicken, Green Beans & Snow Peas Stir Fry

Serves 2

Ingredients - Allergies: SF, GF, DF, EF
- 1/2 pound chicken • 1 cup sliced green beans
- 1/2 cup sliced snow peas
- 1 Tbsp. coconut oil

Instructions

Marinade chicken in a Superfoods marinade. Stir fry drained chicken in coconut oil for few minutes, add green beans and snow peas and stir fry for 2 more minutes. Add the rest of the marinade and stir fry for a minute. Serve with brown rice or quinoa.

Mushrooms, Snow Peas & Broccoli Stir Fry

Serves 2

Ingredients - Allergies: SF, GF, DF, EF

- 1/2 pound mushrooms • 1 cup sliced Broccoli
- 1/2 cup sliced snow peas
- 1 Tbsp. coconut oil

Instructions

Marinade mushrooms in a Superfoods marinade. Stir fry drained mushrooms in coconut oil for few minutes, add broccoli and snow peas and stir fry for 2 more minutes. Add the rest of the marinade and stir fry for a minute. Serve with brown rice or quinoa.

Yellow Squash, Zucchini, Eggplant & Onions Stir Fry

Serves 2

Ingredients - Allergies: SF, GF, DF, EF

- 1/4 pound zucchini
- 1/4 pound yellow squash
- 1 cup sliced eggplant
- 1/2 cup sliced onions
- 1 Tbsp. coconut oil

Instructions

Marinade eggplant, squash and zucchini in a Superfoods marinade. Stir fry drained veggies in coconut oil for few minutes, add onions and stir fry for 2 more minutes. Add the rest of the marinade and stir fry for a minute. Serve with brown rice or quinoa.

Shiitake, GreenPeppers & Bamboo Shoots Stir Fry

Serves 2

Ingredients - Allergies: SF, GF, DF, EF

- 1/2 pound shiitake • 1/2 cup sliced black mushrooms
- 1/2 cup sliced green peppers
- 1/2 cup sliced dried bamboo shoots
- 1 Tbsp. coconut oil

Instructions

Marinade shiitake in a Superfoods marinade. Stir fry drained shiitake in coconut oil for few minutes, add broccoli and water chestnuts and stir fry for 2 more minutes. Add the rest of the marinade and stir fry for a minute. Serve with brown rice or quinoa.

Shiitake, Shrimp & Asparagus Stir Fry

Serves 2

Ingredients - Allergies: SF, GF, DF, EF
- 1/2 pound shrimp • 1 cup sliced Asparagus
- 1/2 cup sliced shiitake
- 1 Tbsp. coconut oil

Instructions

Marinade shrimp in a Superfoods marinade. Stir fry drained shrimp in coconut oil for few minutes, add asparagus and shiitake and stir fry for 2 more minutes. Add the rest of the marinade and stir fry for a minute. Serve with brown rice or quinoa.

Shrimp, Celery & Garlic Stir Fry

Serves 2

Ingredients - Allergies: SF, GF, DF, EF
- 1/2 pound shrimp • 1 + 1/2 cup sliced Celery
- 2 minced garlic cloves
- 1 Tbsp. coconut oil

Instructions

Marinade shrimp in a Superfoods marinade. Stir fry drained shrimp in coconut oil for few minutes, add celery and garlic and stir fry for 2 more minutes. Add the rest of the marinade and stir fry for a minute. Serve with brown rice or quinoa.

Squid, Shrimp, Celery & Bitter Gourd Stir Fry

Serves 2

Ingredients - Allergies: SF, GF, DF, EF
- 1/4 pound shrimp
- 1/4 pound squid • 1 cup sliced Celery
- 1/2 cup sliced bitter gourd
- 1 Tbsp. coconut oil

Instructions

Marinade shrimp and squid in a Superfoods marinade. Stir fry drained shrimp and squid in coconut oil for few minutes, add celery and biter gourd and stir fry for 2 more minutes. Add the rest of the marinade and stir fry for a minute. Serve with brown rice or quinoa.

Sechuan Beef, Celery, Carrot & Chili Sauce Stir Fry

Serves 2

Ingredients - Allergies: SF, GF, DF, EF
- 1/2 pound beef • 1 cup sliced celery
- 1/2 cup sliced carrot
- 1 Tbsp. coconut oil

Instructions

Marinade beef in a Superfoods marinade and chili sauce. Stir fry drained beef in coconut oil for few minutes, add celery and carrot and stir fry for 2 more minutes. Add the rest of the marinade and stir fry for a minute. Serve with brown rice or quinoa.

Asparagus, Yellow Peppers & Tomato Stir Fry

Serves 2

Ingredients - Allergies: SF, GF, DF, EF
- 1/2 pound asparagus • 1 cup sliced Yellow peppers
- 1 cup chopped tomato
- 1 Tbsp. coconut oil

Instructions

Marinade asparagus in a Superfoods marinade. Stir fry drained asparagus in coconut oil for 7-8 minutes, add peppers and tomato and stir fry for 2 more minutes. Add the rest of the marinade and stir fry for a minute. Serve with brown rice or quinoa.

Beef, Sprouts, Yellow Peppers & Snow Peas Stir Fry

Serves 2

Ingredients - Allergies: SF, GF, DF, EF
- 1/2 pound beef • 1 cup sprouts
- 1 cup Yellow peppers
- 1/2 cup snow peas
- 1 Tbsp. coconut oil

Instructions

Marinade beef in a Superfoods marinade. Stir fry drained beef in coconut oil for few minutes, add yellow peppers and snow peas and stir fry for 2 more minutes. Add sprouts and the rest of the marinade and stir fry for a minute. Serve with brown rice or quinoa.

Bok Choy, Almonds, Onions & Sesame Stir Fry

Serves 2

Ingredients - Allergies: SF, GF, DF, EF
- 1/2 pound bok choy • 1 + ½ cup sliced onions
- 3 Tbsp. almond slices
- 1 Tbsp. sesame seeds
- 1 Tbsp. coconut oil

Instructions

Marinade bok choy in a Superfoods marinade. Stir fry drained bok choy and onions in coconut oil for few minutes, add almond and sesame seeds and stir fry for 2 more minutes. Add the rest of the marinade and stir fry for a minute. Serve with brown rice or quinoa.

Broccoli, Turkey Breast & Carrots Stir Fry

Serves 2

Ingredients - Allergies: SF, GF, DF, EF
- 1/2 pound turkey breast, cubed • 1 cup sliced broccoli
- 3/4 cup sliced carrots
- 1 Tbsp. coconut oil

Instructions

Marinade turkey in a Superfoods marinade. Stir fry drained turkey in coconut oil for few minutes, add carrot and broccoli and stir fry for 2 more minutes. Add the rest of the marinade and stir fry for a minute. Serve with brown rice or quinoa.

Broccolini, Zucchini, Tomatoes & Onions Stir Fry

Serves 2

Ingredients - Allergies: SF, GF, DF, EF
- 1/2 pound broccolini • 1 cup sliced zucchini
- 3/4 cup sliced onions
- 3/4 cup chopped tomato
- 1 Tbsp. coconut oil

Instructions

Marinade broccolini in a Superfoods marinade. Stir fry drained broccolini in coconut oil for few minutes, add zucchini and onions and stir fry for 2 more minutes. Add tomatoes and the rest of the marinade and stir fry for a minute. Serve with brown rice or quinoa.

Chicken, Green Beans & Snow Peas Stir Fry

Serves 2

Ingredients - Allergies: SF, GF, DF, EF
- 1/2 pound chicken • 1 cup halved asparagus
- 1 cup snow peas
- 1 Tbsp. sliced green onions
- 1 Tbsp. coconut oil

Instructions

Marinade chicken in a Superfoods marinade. Stir fry drained chicken and asparagus in coconut oil for few minutes, add snow peas and stir fry for 4-5 more minutes. Add the rest of the marinade and stir fry for a minute. Sprinkle with green onions. Serve with brown rice or quinoa.

Eggplant, Mushrooms, Carrots & Snow Peas Stir Fry

Serves 2

Ingredients - Allergies: SF, GF, DF, EF
- 1/2 pound eggplant • 1 + 1/2 cup mushrooms
- 1/2 cup sliced carrot
- 1 cup sliced snow peas
- 1 minced garlic clove
- 1 Tbsp. coconut oil

Instructions

Marinade eggplant in a Superfoods marinade. Stir fry drained eggplant in coconut oil for few minutes, add carrot, snow peas and garlic and stir fry for 2 more minutes. Add the rest of the marinade and stir fry for a minute. Serve with brown rice or quinoa.

Kale, Baby Corn & Shrimp Stir Fry

Serves 2

Ingredients - Allergies: SF, GF, DF, EF
- 1/2 pound shrimp • 1 + 1/2 cup sliced Kale
- 1 cup baby corn
- 1 Tbsp. coconut oil

Instructions

Marinade shrimp in a Superfoods marinade. Stir fry drained shrimp in coconut oil for few minutes, add kale and baby corn and stir fry for 2 more minutes. Add the rest of the marinade and stir fry for a minute. Serve with brown rice or quinoa.

Lamb, Baby Corn, Red Peppers & Green Beans Stir Fry

Serves 2

Ingredients - Allergies: SF, GF, DF, EF
- 1/2 pound lamb • 1 cup sliced red peppers
- 3/4 cup sliced green beans
- 1/2 cup baby corn
- 1 Tbsp. coconut oil

Instructions

Marinade lamb in a Superfoods marinade. Stir fry drained lamb in coconut oil for few minutes, add green beans, baby corn and peppers and stir fry for 2 more minutes. Add the rest of the marinade and stir fry for a minute. Serve with brown rice or quinoa.

Minced Pork, Mushrooms & Red Peppers Stir Fry

Serves 2

Ingredients - Allergies: SF, GF, DF, EF
- 1/2 pound minced pork meat • 1 + 1/2 cup sliced Mushrooms
- 3/4 cup sliced red peppers
- 3/4 cup sliced green peppers
- 1 Tbsp. coconut oil

Instructions

Stir fry minced pork meat in coconut oil for few minutes, add red and green peppers and mushrooms and stir fry for 2 more minutes. Add the superfoods marinade and stir fry for a minute. Serve with brown rice or quinoa.

Brussel Sprouts, Broccoli, Chicken & Leeks Stir Fry

Serves 2

Ingredients - Allergies: SF, GF, DF, EF
- 1/2 pound chicken • 1 cup sliced Brussels sprouts
- 1 cup broccoli
- 1/2 cup sliced leeks
- 1 Tbsp. coconut oil

Instructions

Marinade chicken in a Superfoods marinade. Stir fry drained chicken and Brussels sprouts in coconut oil for few minutes, add leeks and broccoli and stir fry for 4-5 more minutes. Add the rest of the marinade and stir fry for a minute. Serve with brown rice or quinoa.

Chicken, Cashews & Green Beans Stir Fry

Serves 2

Ingredients - Allergies: SF, GF, DF, EF
- 1/2 pound chicken • 1 cup Green beans
- 1 cup cashews
- 1 Tbsp. coconut oil

Instructions

Marinade chicken in a Superfoods marinade. Stir fry drained chicken and green beans in coconut oil for few minutes, add cashews and stir fry for 4-5 more minutes. Add the rest of the marinade and stir fry for a minute. Serve with brown rice or quinoa.

Lamb, Shallots, Red Peppers & Green Onions Stir Fry

Serves 2

Ingredients - Allergies: SF, GF, DF, EF
- 1/2 pound lamb • 1/2 cup green peppers
- 1 cup red peppers
- 1/2 cup shallots
- 2 Tbsp. sliced green onions
- 1 Tbsp. coconut oil

Instructions

Marinade lamb in a Superfoods marinade. Stir fry drained lamb in coconut oil for few minutes, add shallots, green peppers and red peppers and stir fry for 4-5 more minutes. Add the rest of the marinade and stir fry for a minute. Sprinkle with green onions. Serve with brown rice or quinoa.

Mixed Seafood, Green Beans & Sprouts Stir Fry

Serves 2

Ingredients - Allergies: SF, GF, DF, EF
- 1/2 pound mixed seafood • 1 cup green beans
- 1 cup sprouts
- 1 half of the carrot, sliced
- 1 Tbsp. coconut oil

Instructions

Marinade seafood in a Superfoods marinade. Stir fry drained seafood and green beans in coconut oil for few minutes, add carrot and stir fry for 4-5 more minutes. Add the rest of the marinade and sprouts and stir fry for a minute. Serve with brown rice or quinoa.

Pork, Mushrooms & Green Beans Stir Fry

Serves 2

Ingredients - Allergies: SF, GF, DF, EF
- 1/2 pound pork • 1/2 cup red peppers
- 1 cup green beans
- 1 cup mushrooms
- 1 Tbsp. coconut oil

Instructions

Marinade pork in a Superfoods marinade. Stir fry drained pork and green beans in coconut oil for few minutes, add red peppers and mushrooms and stir fry for 4-5 more minutes. Add the rest of the marinade and stir fry for a minute. Serve with brown rice or quinoa.

Prawns & Snow Peas Stir Fry

Serves 2

Ingredients - Allergies: SF, GF, DF, EF
- 1/2 pound prawns • 2 cups snow peas
- 1 Tbsp. sliced green onions
- 1 Tbsp. coconut oil

Instructions

Marinade prawns in a Superfoods marinade. Stir fry drained prawns in coconut oil for few minutes, add snow peas and stir fry for 4-5 more minutes. Add the rest of the marinade and stir fry for a minute. Sprinkle with green onions. Serve with brown rice or quinoa.

Red Peppers, Yellow Peppers & Olives Stir Fry

Serves 2

Ingredients - Allergies: SF, GF, DF, EF
- 1 cup red peppers
- 1 cup green peppers
- 1 cup yellow peppers
- 1/2 cup carrot
- 1 rosemary sprig
- 1 Tbsp. basil leaves
- 1/2 cup olives
- 1 Tbsp. coconut oil

Instructions

Marinade all 3 types of peppers in a Superfoods marinade. Stir fry drained peppers and carrot in coconut oil for few minutes, add olives and rosemary and stir fry for 4-5 more minutes. Add the rest of the marinade and basil stir fry for a minute. Serve with brown rice or quinoa.

Spinach, Prawns & Water Chestnut Stir Fry

Serves 2

Ingredients - Allergies: SF, GF, DF, EF
- 1/2 pound prawns • 1 cup sliced water chestnut
- 1 cup spinach
- 1 Tbsp. coconut oil

Instructions

Marinade prawns in a Superfoods marinade. Stir fry drained prawns and water chestnut in coconut oil for 4-5 more minutes. Add the rest of the marinade, spinach and stir fry for a minute. Serve with brown rice or quinoa.

Squid, Shrimp, Mussels & Green Beans Stir Fry

Serves 2

Ingredients - Allergies: SF, GF, DF, EF
- 1/2 pound Squid, shrimp and mussels each • 1 cup green beans
- 1/2 cup carrots
- 2 Tbsp. basil leaves
- 1 Tbsp. coconut oil

Instructions

Marinade squid, shrimp and mussels in a Superfoods marinade. Stir fry drained squid, shrimp and mussels and green beans in coconut oil for few minutes, add carrot and stir fry for 4-5 more minutes. Add the rest of the marinade and stir fry for a minute. Sprinkle with basil leaves and mix. Serve with brown rice or quinoa.

Water Chestnut, Chicken & Bok Choy Stir Fry

Serves 2

Ingredients - Allergies: SF, GF, DF, EF
- 1/2 pound chicken • 1 cup sliced water chestnuts
- 1 cup sliced carrot
- 1/2 cup sliced bok choy
- 1 Tbsp. coconut oil

Instructions

Marinade chicken in a Superfoods marinade. Stir fry drained chicken and water chestnut in coconut oil for few minutes, add carrot and stir fry for 4-5 more minutes. Add the rest of the marinade and stir fry for a minute. Sprinkle with green onions. Serve with brown rice or quinoa.

Baby Corn, Bok Choy, Onion & Beef Stir Fry

Serves 2

Ingredients - Allergies: SF, GF, DF, EF
- 1/2 pound beef stripes • 1 cup sliced bok choy
- 1/2 cup baby corn
- 1/2 cup onions
- 1 Tbsp. coconut oil

Instructions

Marinade beef in a Superfoods marinade. Stir fry drained beef and baby corn in coconut oil for 4-5 more minutes. Add the rest of the marinade, onion and bok choy and stir fry for a minute. Serve with brown rice or quinoa.

Bok Choy, Chicken, Snow Peas & Mushrooms Stir Fry

Serves 2

Ingredients - Allergies: SF, GF, DF, EF
- 1/2 pound chicken • 1 cup sliced bok choy
- 1/2 cup snow peas
- 1/2 cup mushrooms
- 1 Tbsp. coconut oil

Instructions

Marinade chicken in a Superfoods marinade. Stir fry drained chicken and snow peas in coconut oil for 4-5 more minutes. Add the rest of the marinade, mushrooms and stir fry for a minute. Serve with brown rice or quinoa.

Broccoli, Green Onions & Red Peppers Stir Fry

Serves 2

Ingredients - Allergies: SF, GF, DF, EF
- 1/2 pound broccoli, with stalks peeled • 1 cup red peppers
- 1 cup green onions
- 1 Tbsp. coconut oil

Instructions

Marinade peeled and sliced broccoli stalks in a Superfoods marinade. Stir fry drained broccoli stalks, broccoli florets and red peppers in coconut oil for 4-5 more minutes. Add the rest of the marinade, green onions and stir fry for a minute. Serve with brown rice or quinoa.

Leeks & Pork Fry

Serves 2

Ingredients - Allergies: SF, GF, DF, EF
- 1/2 pound pork • 2 cups diagonally sliced leeks
- 1/2 cup celery
- 1 Tbsp. coconut oil

Instructions

Marinade pork in a Superfoods marinade. Stir fry drained pork and leeks in coconut oil for 4-5 more minutes. Add the rest of the marinade, celery and stir fry for a minute. Serve with brown rice or quinoa.

Fennel, Bok Choy, Red Pepper & Celery Stir Fry

Serves 2

Ingredients - Allergies: SF, GF, DF, EF
- 1 cup sliced celery • 1 cup sliced fennel bulb
- 1/2 cup sliced red peppers
- 1 cup sliced bok choy
- 1 Tbsp. coconut oil

Instructions

Marinade fennel in a Superfoods marinade. Stir fry drained fennel and celery in coconut oil for 4-5 more minutes. Add the rest of the marinade, bok choy and red peppers and stir fry for a minute. Serve with brown rice or quinoa.

Fish, Wood Ear Mushrooms & Green Peas Stir Fry

Serves 2

Ingredients - Allergies: SF, GF, DF, EF
- 1/2 pound fish filets (e.g. tilapia, cod, sole, flounder) • 1 cup wood ear mushrooms, soaked in water for 30 minutes
- 1/2 cup green peas
- 1 Tbsp. coconut oil

Instructions

Marinade fish in a Superfoods marinade. Stir fry drained fish and green peas in coconut oil for 4-5 more minutes. Add the rest of the marinade, mushrooms and stir fry for a minute. Serve with brown rice or quinoa.

Fish, Bok Choy, Onions & Tomato Stir Fry

Serves 2

Ingredients - Allergies: SF, GF, DF, EF
- 1/2 pound fish filets (e.g. tilapia, cod, sole, flounder) • 1 cup sliced bok choy
- 1/2 cup tomato
- 1/2 cup onions
- 1 Tbsp. coconut oil

Instructions

Marinade fish in a Superfoods marinade. Stir fry drained fish and onions in coconut oil for 4-5 more minutes. Add the rest of the marinade, bok choy and tomato and stir fry for a minute. Serve with brown rice or quinoa.

Green Garlic, Pork, Ginger & Celery Stir Fry

Serves 2

Ingredients - Allergies: SF, GF, DF, EF
- 1/2 pound pork • 1 cup sliced green garlic
- 1 Tbsp. minced ginger
- 1 cup celery
- 1 Tbsp. coconut oil

Instructions

Marinade pork in a Superfoods marinade. Stir fry drained pork and green garlic in coconut oil for 4-5 more minutes. Add the rest of the marinade, ginger and celery and stir fry for a minute. Serve with brown rice or quinoa.

Kale, Beef, Bok Choy & Green Garlic Stir Fry

Serves 2

Ingredients - Allergies: SF, GF, DF, EF
- 1/2 pound beef • 1 cup sliced bok choy
- 1 cup sliced kale
- 1/2 cup sliced green garlic
- 1 Tbsp. coconut oil

Instructions

Marinade beef in a Superfoods marinade. Stir fry drained beef, green garlic and kale in coconut oil for 4-5 more minutes. Add the rest of the marinade, bok choy and stir fry for a minute. Serve with brown rice or quinoa.

Lamb, Broccoli, Mushrooms & Onions Stir Fry

Serves 2
Ingredients - Allergies: SF, GF, DF, EF
- 1/2 pound lamb • 1 cup broccoli
- 1 cup mushrooms
- 1/2 cup onions
- 1 Tbsp. coconut oil

Instructions
Marinade lamb in a Superfoods marinade. Stir fry drained lamb and broccoli in coconut oil for 4-5 more minutes. Add the rest of the marinade, onions and mushrooms and stir fry for a minute. Serve with brown rice or quinoa.

Veal, Bok Choy & Pine Nuts Stir Fry

Serves 2
Ingredients - Allergies: SF, GF, DF, EF
- 1/2 pound veal • 2 cups bok choy
- 1/2 cup onions
- 1/2 cup pine nuts
- 1 Tbsp. coconut oil

Instructions
Marinade veal in a Superfoods marinade. Stir fry drained veal and onions in coconut oil for 3-4 more minutes. Add the rest of the marinade, pine nuts and bok choy and stir fry for 3 minutes more. Serve with brown rice or quinoa.

Chicken, Water Chestnut & Green Onions Stir Fry

Serves 2
Ingredients - Allergies: SF, GF, DF, EF
- 1/2 pound chicken breast • 1/2 cup green onions
- 1/2 cup water chestnut
- 1/2 cup carrot
- 1/4 Tsp. chili flakes
- 1/2 cup celery
- 1 Tbsp. coconut oil

Instructions
Marinade chicken breast in a Superfoods marinade and chili flakes. Stir fry drained chicken, carrot and celery in coconut oil for 4-5 more minutes. Add the rest of the marinade, green onions and water chestnuts and stir fry for 2 minutes more. Serve with brown rice or quinoa.

Chicken, Snow Peas, Carrots & Peppers Stir Fry

Serves 2

Ingredients - Allergies: SF, GF, DF, EF
- 1/2 pound chicken • 1/2 cup snow peas
- 1/2 cup green peas
- 1/2 cup red peppers
- 1/2 cup carrots
- 1/2 cup onions
- 1 Tbsp. coconut oil

Instructions

Marinade chicken in a Superfoods marinade. Stir fry drained chicken, green peas and carrot in coconut oil for 4-5 more minutes. Add the rest of the marinade, onions, snow peas and red peppers and stir fry for a minute. Serve with brown rice or quinoa.

Chicken Dark Meat & Red Peppers Stir Fry

Serves 2

Ingredients - Allergies: SF, GF, DF, EF
- 1/2 pound chicken dark meat • 2 cups red peppers
- 1/2 cup onions
- 1 Tbsp. coconut oil

Instructions

Marinade chicken in a Superfoods marinade. Stir fry drained chicken and red peppers in coconut oil for 4-5 more minutes. Add the rest of the marinade and onions and stir fry for a minute. Serve with brown rice or quinoa.

Fennel, Green Peppers & Veal Stir Fry

Serves 2

Ingredients - Allergies: SF, GF, DF, EF
- 1/2 pound veal • 1 cup sliced fennel bulb
- 1 cup sliced green peppers
- 1/2 cup onions
- 1 Tbsp. coconut oil

Instructions

Marinade veal in a Superfoods marinade. Stir fry drained veal and fennel in coconut oil for 4-5 more minutes. Add the rest of the marinade, onions and green peppers and stir fry for a minute. Serve with brown rice or quinoa.

Pork Belly & Pumpkin Stir Fry

Serves 2
Ingredients - Allergies: SF, GF, DF, EF
- 1/2 pound pork belly • 2 cups pumpkin
- 1/2 cup green onions
- 1 Tbsp. coconut oil

Instructions
Marinade pork in a Superfoods marinade. Stir fry drained pork and pumpkin in coconut oil for 7-8 more minutes. Add the rest of the marinade and green onions and stir fry for a minute. Serve with brown rice or quinoa.

Pork, Peppers & Mushrooms Stir Fry

Serves 2
Ingredients - Allergies: SF, GF, DF, EF
- 1/2 pound pork • 1/2 cup red peppers
- 1/2 cup green peppers
- 1 cup mushrooms
- 1/2 cup onions
- 1 Tbsp. coconut oil

Instructions
Marinade pork in a Superfoods marinade. Stir fry drained pork and peppers in coconut oil for 4-5 more minutes. Add the rest of the marinade, onions and mushrooms and stir fry for a minute. Serve with brown rice or quinoa.

Kale & Pumpkin Stir Fry

Serves 2
Ingredients - Allergies: SF, GF, DF, EF
- 1/2 pound Pumpkin • 2 cups kale
- 1/2 cup onions
- 1 Tbsp. coconut oil

Instructions
Marinade pumpkin in a Superfoods marinade. Stir fry drained pumpkin in coconut oil for 4-5 more minutes. Add the rest of the marinade, onions and kale and stir fry for 2 minutes more. Serve with brown rice or quinoa.

Cauliflower & Green Onions Stir Fry

Serves 2

Ingredients - Allergies: SF, GF, DF, EF
- 1 pound cauliflower • 1 cup green onions
- 1/2 tsp. chili flakes
- 1/2 cup onions
- 1 lime slice
- 1 Tbsp. coconut oil

Instructions

Marinade cauliflower in a Superfoods marinade and chili flakes. Stir fry drained cauliflower in coconut oil for 4-5 more minutes. Add the rest of the marinade, green onions and onions and stir fry for a minute. Decorate with lime slice and serve with brown rice or quinoa.

Veal, Asparagus & Chinese Celery Stir Fry

Serves 2

Ingredients - Allergies: SF, GF, DF, EF
- 1/2 pound veal • 1 cup Asparagus
- 1 cup Chinese celery
- 1/2 cup onions
- 1 Tbsp. coconut oil

Instructions

Marinade veal in a Superfoods marinade. Stir fry drained veal and asparagus in coconut oil for 4-5 more minutes. Add the rest of the marinade, onions and Chinese celery and stir fry for a minute. Serve with brown rice or quinoa.

Calamari & Green Peas Stir Fry

Serves 2

Ingredients - Allergies: SF, GF, DF, EF
- 1/2 pound calamari (squid rings) • 2 cups Green Peas
- 1/2 cup sliced onions
- 1 Tbsp. coconut oil *Instructions*

Marinade calamari in a Superfoods marinade. Stir fry drained calamari and green peas in coconut oil for few minutes, add onions and stir fry for 2 more minutes. Add the rest of the marinade and stir fry for a minute. Serve with brown rice or quinoa.

Chicken Breast & Snow Peas Stir Fry

Serves 2
Ingredients - Allergies: SF, GF, DF, EF
- 1/2-pound chicken breast • 2 cups Snow Peas
- 1/2 cup sliced red peppers
- 1/2 cup Baby Corn
- 1 Tbsp. coconut oil *Instructions*

Marinade chicken in a Superfoods marinade. Stir fry drained chicken in coconut oil for few minutes, add all vegetables and stir fry for 2 more minutes. Add the rest of the marinade and stir fry for a minute. Serve with brown rice or quinoa.

Chicken, Broccoli & Cauliflower Stir Fry

Serves 2
Ingredients - Allergies: SF, GF, DF, EF
- 1/2-pound chicken • 1 cup Cauliflower
- 1/2 cup sliced Carrots
- 1 cup Broccoli
- 1 Tbsp. chopped onion
- 1 Tbsp. coconut oil *Instructions*

Marinade chicken in a Superfoods marinade. Stir fry drained chicken in coconut oil for few minutes, add all vegetables and stir fry for 2 more minutes. Add the rest of the marinade and stir fry for a minute. Serve with brown rice or quinoa.

Chicken & Celery Stir Fry

Serves 2
Ingredients - Allergies: SF, GF, DF, EF
- 1/2-pound chicken • 2 cups Celery, diagonally sliced
- 1/2 cup sliced Carrots
- 1 Tbsp. coconut oil *Instructions*

Marinade chicken in a Superfoods marinade. Stir fry drained chicken in coconut oil for few minutes, add all vegetables and stir fry for 2 more minutes. Add the rest of the marinade and stir fry for a minute. Serve with brown rice or quinoa over bed of lettuce.

Chicken, Peppers & Cashew Stir Fry

Serves 2

Ingredients - Allergies: SF, GF, DF, EF
- 1/2-pound chicken • 1 cup Red Peppers
- 1 cup sliced Green Peppers
- 1/2 cup Cashew
- 1 Tbsp. coconut oil *Instructions*

Marinade chicken in a Superfoods marinade. Stir fry drained chicken in coconut oil for few minutes, add all vegetables and cashew and stir fry for 2 more minutes. Add the rest of the marinade and stir fry for a minute. Serve with brown rice or quinoa.

Kale & 2 Mushrooms Stir Fry

Serves 2

Ingredients - Allergies: SF, GF, DF, EF
- 1/2-pound shiitake and Portobello mushrooms • 2 cups Kale
- 1/2 cup sliced onions
- 1 Tbsp. coconut oil *Instructions*

Marinade shiitake in a Superfoods marinade. Stir fry drained shiitake and kale in coconut oil for few minutes, add all other vegetables and stir fry for 2 more minutes. Add the rest of the marinade and stir fry for a minute. Serve with brown rice or quinoa.

Kale, Carrot & Green Peas Stir Fry

Serves 2

Ingredients - Allergies: SF, GF, DF, EF
- 1/2 pound green peas • 2 cups Kale
- 1/2 cup sliced Carrots
- 1/2 cup onion
- 1 Tbsp. coconut oil *Instructions*

Marinade green peas in a Superfoods marinade. Stir fry drained green peas and kale in coconut oil for few minutes, add all vegetables and stir fry for 2 more minutes. Add the rest of the marinade and stir fry for a minute. Serve with brown rice or quinoa.

Pepper Steak Stir Fry

Serves 2

Ingredients - Allergies: SF, GF, DF, EF
- 1/2-pound steak • 1 cup Red Peppers
- 1/2 cup sliced green onions
- 1/2 cup sliced carrot
- 1 Tbsp. black pepper
- 1 Tbsp. coconut oil *Instructions*

Marinade steak in a Superfoods marinade and black pepper. Stir fry drained steak in coconut oil for few minutes, add all vegetables and stir fry for 2 more minutes. Add the rest of the marinade and stir fry for a minute. Serve with brown rice or quinoa.

Shrimp, Carrot, Red Peppers & Green Onion Stir Fry

Serves 2

Ingredients - Allergies: SF, GF, DF, EF
- 1/2-pound shrimp • 1 cup red peppers
- 1/2 cup sliced Carrots
- 1/2 cup sliced green onions
- 1 Tbsp. coconut oil *Instructions*

Marinade shrimp in a Superfoods marinade. Stir fry drained shrimp in coconut oil for few minutes, add all vegetables and stir fry for 2 more minutes. Add the rest of the marinade and stir fry for a minute. Serve with brown rice or quinoa.

Veal Szechuan Stir Fry

Serves 2

Ingredients - Allergies: SF, GF, DF, EF
- 1/2-pound veal • 1/2 cup red peppers
- 1/2 cup sliced Carrots
- 1/2 cup green peppers
- ½ cup onions
- 1 Tsp. Szechuan peppercorns, ground
- 1 Tsp. red pepper flakes
- 1 Tbsp. coconut oil *Instructions*

Marinade veal in a Superfoods marinade, Szechuan ground peppercorns and red pepper flakes. Stir fry drained veal in coconut oil for few minutes, add all vegetables and stir fry for 2 more minutes. Add the rest of the marinade and stir fry for a minute. Serve with brown rice or quinoa.

Beef, Asparagus & Enokitake Stir Fry

Serves 2

Ingredients - Allergies: SF, GF, DF, EF
- 1/2 pound beef • 1 + 1/2 cups sliced asparagus
- 1/2 cup sliced Onions
- 1/2 cup sliced Enokitake mushrooms (optional shiitake)
- 1 Tbsp. oil *Instructions*

Marinade beef in a Superfoods marinade. Stir fry drained beef in coconut oil for few minutes, add all vegetables and stir fry for 2 more minutes. Add the rest of the marinade and stir fry for a minute. Serve with brown rice or quinoa.

Beef, Celery, Zucchini, Green Onions & Broccoli Stir Fry

Serves 2

Ingredients - Allergies: SF, GF, DF, EF
- 1/2-pound beef • 1/2 cups sliced broccoli
- 1/2 cup sliced green Onions
- 1/2 cup sliced zucchini
- 1/2 cup sliced celery
- 1 Tbsp. oil *Instructions*

Marinade beef in a Superfoods marinade. Stir fry drained beef in coconut oil for few minutes, add all vegetables and stir fry for 2 more minutes. Add the rest of the marinade and stir fry for a minute. Serve with brown rice or quinoa.

Carrot, Broccoli, Snow Peas, Chicken & Water Chestnut Stir Fry

Serves 2

Ingredients - Allergies: SF, GF, DF, EF
- 1/2-pound chicken • 1 cup sliced carrot
- 1/2 cup sliced Onions
- 1/2 cup sliced snow peas
- 1/2 cup sliced water chestnut
- 1/2 cup sliced broccoli
- 1 Tbsp. oil *Instructions*

Marinade chicken in a Superfoods marinade. Stir fry drained chicken in coconut oil for few minutes, add all vegetables and stir fry for 2 more minutes. Add the rest of the marinade and stir fry for a minute. Serve with brown rice or quinoa.

Chicken, Leeks, Red Peppers & Napa Cabbage Stir Fry

Serves 2

Ingredients - Allergies: SF, GF, DF, EF
- 1/2-pound chicken • 1/2 cups sliced Napa cabbage
- 1/2 cup sliced leeks
- 1/4 cup cashews
- 1 Tbsp. oil *Instructions*

Marinade chicken in a Superfoods marinade. Stir fry drained chicken in coconut oil for few minutes, add all vegetables and stir fry for 2 more minutes. Add the rest of the marinade and stir fry for a minute. Serve with brown rice or quinoa.

Cucumber, Shiitake, Shrimp & Garlic Stir Fry

Serves 2

Ingredients - Allergies: SF, GF, DF, EF
- 1/2-pound shrimp • 1 cup sliced peeled and sliced cucumber
- 1/2 cup sliced Onions
- 1 cup sliced Shiitake
- 1 Tbsp. oil *Instructions*

Marinade shrimp in a Superfoods marinade. Stir fry drained shrimp in coconut oil for few minutes, add onions and shiitake and stir fry for 2 more minutes. Add the rest of the marinade and cucumber and stir fry for a minute. Serve with brown rice or quinoa.

Lamb, Broccoli, Carrot & Cauliflower Stir Fry

Serves 2

Ingredients - Allergies: SF, GF, DF, EF
- 1/2-pound lamb • 1/2 cup sliced cauliflower
- 1/2 cup sliced Onions
- 1/2 cup sliced broccoli
- 1/2 cup sliced carrot
- 1 Tbsp. oil *Instructions*

Marinade lamb in a Superfoods marinade. Stir fry drained lamb in coconut oil for few minutes, add all vegetables and stir fry for 2 more minutes. Add the rest of the marinade and stir fry for a minute. Serve with brown rice or quinoa.

Shrimps, Green Beans, Celery & Carrots Stir Fry

Serves 2

Ingredients - Allergies: SF, GF, DF, EF
- 1/2-pound shrimp • 1/2 cup sliced green beans
- 1/2 cup sliced Onions
- 1/2 cup sliced carrot
- 1/2 cup sliced celery
- 1 Tbsp. oil *Instructions*

Marinade shrimp in a Superfoods marinade. Stir fry drained shrimp in coconut oil for few minutes, add all vegetables and stir fry for 2 more minutes. Add the rest of the marinade and stir fry for a minute. Serve with brown rice or quinoa.

Water Chestnut, Broccoli, Carrots, Snow Peas & Shrimp Stir Fry

Serves 2

Ingredients - Allergies: SF, GF, DF, EF
- 1/2-pound shrimp • 1/2 cup sliced water chestnut
- 1/2 cup sliced Onions
- 1/2 cup sliced carrots
- 1/2 cup sliced snow peas
- 1/2 cup sliced broccoli
- 1 Tbsp. oil *Instructions*

Marinade shrimp in a Superfoods marinade. Stir fry drained shrimp in coconut oil for few minutes, add all vegetables and stir fry for 2 more minutes. Add the rest of the marinade and stir fry for a minute. Serve with brown rice or quinoa.

Yellow Squash, Broccoli, Snow Peas & Shiitake Stir Fry

Serves 2

Ingredients - Allergies: SF, GF, DF, EF
- 1/2-pound chicken • 1/2 cup sliced yellow squash
- 1 cup sliced broccoli
- 1/2 cup sliced snow peas
- 1/2 cup sliced shiitake
- 1 Tbsp. oil *Instructions*

Marinade chicken in a Superfoods marinade. Stir fry drained chicken in coconut oil for few minutes, add all vegetables and stir fry for 2 more minutes. Add the rest of the marinade and stir fry for a minute. Serve with brown rice or quinoa.

Zucchini, Green Beans, Leeks & Shrimp Stir Fry

Serves 2

Ingredients - Allergies: SF, GF, DF, EF
- 1/2 pound shrimp • 1 cup sliced zucchini
- 1 cup sliced green beans
- 1/2 cup sliced leeks
- 1 Tbsp. oil *Instructions*

Marinade shrimp in a Superfoods marinade. Stir fry drained shrimp in coconut oil for few minutes, add all vegetables and stir fry for 2 more minutes. Add the rest of the marinade and stir fry for a minute. Serve with brown rice or quinoa.

Asparagus, Snow Peas, Chicken & Green Onions Stir Fry

Serves 2

Ingredients - Allergies: SF, GF, DF, EF
- 1/2 pound cubed chicken • 1 cup sliced asparagus
- 1/2 cup snow peas
- 1/2 cup sliced green onions
- 1 Tsp.oil *Instructions*

Marinade chicken in a Superfoods marinade. Stir fry drained chicken and asparagus in coconut oil for few minutes, add all other vegetables and stir fry for 2 more minutes. Add the rest of the marinade and stir fry for a minute. Serve with brown rice or quinoa.

Asparagus, Water Chestnut & Shrimp Stir Fry

Serves 2

Ingredients - Allergies: SF, GF, DF, EF
- 1/2 pound shrimp • 1 cup sliced asparagus
- 1 cup water chestnut
- 1 Tsp.oil *Instructions*

Marinade shrimp in a Superfoods marinade. Stir fry drained shrimp and asparagus in coconut oil for few minutes, add water chestnut and stir fry for 2 more minutes. Add the rest of the marinade and stir fry for a minute. Serve with brown rice or quinoa.

Baby Bok Choy, Water Chestnut, Asparagus, Chicken & Red Peppers Stir Fry

Serves 2

Ingredients - Allergies: SF, GF, DF, EF
- 1/2 pound cubed chicken • 1/2 cup sliced water chestnut
- 3 baby bok choy
- 1/2 cup sliced asparagus
- 1/2 cup sliced red peppers
- 1 Tsp.oil *Instructions*

Marinade chicken in a Superfoods marinade. Stir fry drained chicken and asparagus in coconut oil for few minutes, add all other vegetables and stir fry for 2 more minutes. Add the rest of the marinade and stir fry for a minute. Serve with brown rice or quinoa.

Baby Carrots, Shrimp, Broccoli & Portobello Stir Fry

Serves 2

Ingredients - Allergies: SF, GF, DF, EF
- 1/2 pound cubed shrimp • 1 cup sliced Portobello mushrooms
- 1/2 cup broccoli
- 1/2 cup baby carrots
- 1 Tsp.oil *Instructions*

Marinade shrimp in a Superfoods marinade. Stir fry drained shrimp in coconut oil for few minutes, add all vegetables and stir fry for 2 more minutes. Add the rest of the marinade and stir fry for a minute. Serve with brown rice or quinoa.

Cauliflower, Beef, Carrot, Broccoli & Mushrooms Stir Fry

Serves 2

Ingredients - Allergies: SF, GF, DF, EF
- 1/2-pound cubed beef • 1/2 cup sliced cauliflower
- 1/2 cup sliced broccoli
- 1/2 cup sliced mushrooms
- 1/2 cup sliced carrots
- 1 Tsp.oil *Instructions*

Marinade beef in a Superfoods marinade. Stir fry drained beef in coconut oil for few minutes, add all vegetables and stir fry for 2 more minutes. Add the rest of the marinade and stir fry for a minute. Serve with brown rice or quinoa.

Cauliflower, Chicken, Broccoli, Cashew & Red Pepper Fry

Serves 2

Ingredients - Allergies: SF, GF, DF, EF
- 1/2 pound cubed chicken • 1 cup sliced broccoli
- 1 cup sliced cauliflower
- 1/2 cup cashew
- 1/2 cup sliced red peppers
- 1 Tsp.oil *Instructions*

Marinade chicken in a Superfoods marinade. Stir fry drained chicken in coconut oil for few minutes, add all vegetables and stir fry for 2 more minutes. Add the rest of the marinade and stir fry for a minute. Serve with brown rice or quinoa.

Green Beans, Shrimp, Sesame, Broccoli, Red Peppers & Portobello Stir Fry

Serves 2

Ingredients - Allergies: SF, GF, DF, EF
- 1/2 pound cubed shrimp • 1 cup sliced green beans
- 1/2 cup broccoli
- 1/4 cup sesame seeds
- 1/2 cup sliced carrots and red peppers
- 1 Tsp.oil *Instructions*

Marinade shrimp in a Superfoods marinade. Stir fry drained shrimp in coconut oil for few minutes, add all vegetables and stir fry for 2 more minutes. Add the rest of the marinade and stir fry for a minute. Serve with brown rice or quinoa.

Green Peppers, Sprouts, Chicken, Mushrooms & Parsley Stir Fry

Serves 2

Ingredients - Allergies: SF, GF, DF, EF
- 1/2 pound cubed chicken • 1 cup sliced green peppers
- 1/2 cup sliced mushrooms
- 1/4 cup chopped parsley
- 1/2 cup sprouts
- 1 Tsp.oil *Instructions*

Marinade chicken in a Superfoods marinade. Stir fry drained chicken in coconut oil for few minutes, add all vegetables and stir fry for 2 more minutes. Add the rest of the marinade and stir fry for a minute. Serve with brown rice or quinoa.

Pork, Red Onions & Red Peppers Stir Fry

Serves 2

Ingredients - Allergies: SF, GF, DF, EF
- 1/2 pound cubed pork • 1 cup sliced red peppers
- 1 cup sliced red onions
- 1 Tsp.oil *Instructions*

Marinade pork in a Superfoods marinade. Stir fry drained pork in coconut oil for few minutes, add all vegetables and stir fry for 2 more minutes. Add the rest of the marinade and stir fry for a minute. Serve with brown rice or quinoa.

Sprouts, Broccoli, Red Peppers, Chicken & Cashew Stir Fry

Serves 2

Ingredients - Allergies: SF, GF, DF, EF
- 1/2 pound cubed chicken • 1 cup sliced broccoli
- 1/2 cup sliced red peppers
- 1/2 cup cashews
- 1/2 cup sprouts
- 1 Tsp.oil *Instructions*

Marinade chicken in a Superfoods marinade. Stir fry drained chicken in coconut oil for few minutes, add all vegetables and stir fry for 2 more minutes. Add the rest of the marinade and stir fry for a minute. Serve with brown rice or quinoa.

Baby Corn, Beef & Ginger Stir Fry

Serves 2

Ingredients - Allergies: SF, GF, DF, EF
- 1/2 pound beef • 2 cups baby corn
- 1 cup sliced onions
- 1 Tbsp. coconut oil
- 2 Tsp. minced ginger

Instructions

Marinade beef in a Superfoods marinade. Stir fry drained beef in coconut oil for few minutes, add ginger, onions and baby corn and stir fry for 2 more minutes. Add the rest of the marinade and stir fry for a minute. Serve with brown rice or quinoa.

Beef, Bok Choy & Red Peppers Stir Fry

Serves 2
Ingredients - Allergies: SF, GF, DF, EF
- 1/2 pound beef • 1 cup sliced bok choy
- 1/2 cup sliced cilantro
- 1/2 cup sliced onions
- 1 Tbsp. coconut oil
- 1/4 cup red peppers

Instructions

Marinade beef in a Superfoods marinade. Stir fry drained beef in coconut oil for few minutes, add onions, bok choy and peppers and stir fry for 2 more minutes. Add the rest of the marinade and cilantro and stir fry for a minute. Serve with brown rice or quinoa.

Cabbage, Carrots, Pork & Almonds Stir Fry

Serves 2
Ingredients - Allergies: SF, GF, DF, EF
- 1/2 pound pork • 2 cups sliced cabbage
- 1/4 cup sliced carrot
- 1/2 cup sliced onions
- 1 Tbsp. coconut oil
- 2 Tbsp. almonds

Instructions

Marinade pork in a Superfoods marinade. Stir fry drained pork in coconut oil for few minutes, add onions, carrots, almonds and cabbage and stir fry for 2 more minutes. Add the rest of the marinade and stir fry for a minute. Serve with brown rice or quinoa.

Carrot, Leeks & Chicken Stir Fry

Serves 2
Ingredients - Allergies: SF, GF, DF, EF
- 1/2 pound chicken • 1 + 1/2 cup sliced leeks
- 1 cup sliced carrots
- 1 Tbsp. coconut oil

Instructions

Marinade chicken in a Superfoods marinade. Stir fry drained chicken in coconut oil for few minutes, add leeks and carrots and stir fry for 2 more minutes. Add the rest of the marinade and stir fry for a minute. Serve with brown rice or quinoa.

Lotus Root, Green Peas, Beef & Carrot Stir Fry

Serves 2

Ingredients - Allergies: SF, GF, DF, EF
- 1/2 pound beef • 1 cup sliced lotus root
- 1/2 cup sliced carrot
- 1/2 cup sliced onions
- 1 Tbsp. coconut oil
- 1/2 green peas

Instructions

Marinade beef in a Superfoods marinade. Stir fry drained beef in coconut oil for few minutes, add all veggies and stir fry for 2 more minutes. Add the rest of the marinade and stir fry for a minute. Serve with brown rice or quinoa.

Shiitake, Bamboo Shoots & Chicken Stir Fry

Serves 2

Ingredients - Allergies: SF, GF, DF, EF
- 1/2 pound chicken • 1 cup sliced bamboo shoots
- 1 cup sliced shiitake
- 1/2 cup sliced onions
- 1 Tbsp. coconut oil
- 2 Tsp. sesame seeds and minced green onions each

Instructions

Marinade chicken in a Superfoods marinade. Stir fry drained chicken in coconut oil for few minutes, add onions, bamboo shoots and shiitake and stir fry for 2 more minutes. Add the rest of the marinade and stir fry for a minute. Decorate with green onions and sesame seeds. Serve with brown rice or quinoa.

Shiitake, Leeks & Chicken Stir Fry

Serves 2

Ingredients - Allergies: SF, GF, DF, EF
- 1/2 pound chicken • 1 + 1/2 cup sliced leeks
- 1 cup sliced shiitake
- 1 Tbsp. coconut oil

Instructions

Marinade chicken in a Superfoods marinade. Stir fry drained chicken in coconut oil for few minutes, add leeks and shiitake and stir fry for 2 more minutes. Add the rest of the marinade and stir fry for a minute. Serve with brown rice or quinoa.

Shrimp, Green Beans, Bok Choy & Carrot Stir Fry

Serves 2
Ingredients - Allergies: SF, GF, DF, EF
- 1/2 pound shrimp • 1 cup sliced green beans
- 1 cup sliced bok choy
- 1/2 cup sliced onions
- 1 Tbsp. coconut oil
- 1/2 carrot

Instructions
Marinade shrimp in a Superfoods marinade. Stir fry drained shrimp in coconut oil for few minutes, add all veggies and stir fry for 2 more minutes. Add the rest of the marinade and stir fry for a minute. Serve with brown rice or quinoa.

Shrimp, Baby Corn & Lotus Root Stir Fry

Serves 2
Ingredients - Allergies: SF, GF, DF, EF
- 1/2 pound shrimp • 1/2 cup sliced baby corn
- 1 cup sliced lotus root
- 1/2 cup sliced onions
- 1 Tbsp. coconut oil
- 1/2 cup sliced shiitake

Instructions
Marinade shrimp in a Superfoods marinade. Stir fry drained shrimp in coconut oil for few minutes, add all veggies and stir fry for 2 more minutes. Add the rest of the marinade and stir fry for a minute. Serve with brown rice or quinoa.

Squid, Red Peppers & Celery Stir Fry

Serves 2
Ingredients - Allergies: SF, GF, DF, EF
- 1/2 pound squid • 1/2 cup sliced red peppers
- 1 + 1/2 cup sliced celery
- 1/2 cup sliced onions
- 1 Tbsp. coconut oil

Instructions
Marinade squid in a Superfoods marinade. Stir fry drained squid in coconut oil for few minutes, add all veggies and stir fry for 2 more minutes. Add the rest of the marinade and stir fry for a minute. Serve with brown rice or quinoa.

Spicy Octopus, Bok Choy & Green Onions Stir Fry

Serves 2

Ingredients - Allergies: SF, GF, DF, EF

- 1/2 pound octopus • 1/4 cup sesame seeds
- 1 + 1/2 cup sliced bok choy
- 1/2 cup sliced green onions
- 1 Tbsp. chili powder (to taste)
- 1 Tbsp. coconut oil

Instructions

Marinade octopus in a Superfoods marinade. Stir fry drained octopus in coconut oil for few minutes, add all veggies and stir fry for 2 more minutes. Add the rest of the marinade and stir fry for a minute. Serve with brown rice or quinoa.

Beef, Mushrooms & Garbanzo Beans Stir Fry

Serves 2

Ingredients - Allergies: SF, GF, DF, EF

- 1/2 pound beef • 1/2 cup drained garbanzo beans
- 1 + 1/2 cup sliced mushrooms
- 1/2 cup sliced onions
- 1 Tbsp. coconut oil

Instructions

Marinade beef in a Superfoods marinade. Stir fry drained beef in coconut oil for few minutes, add all veggies and stir fry for 2 more minutes. Add the rest of the marinade and stir fry for a minute. Serve with brown rice or quinoa.

Pork, Okra& Red Peppers Stir Fry

Serves 2

Ingredients - Allergies: SF, GF, DF, EF

- 1/2 pound pork • 1 cup sliced red peppers
- 1 cup okra
- 1/2 cup sliced mushrooms & zucchini each
- 1 Tbsp. coconut oil

Instructions

Marinade pork in a Superfoods marinade. Stir fry drained pork in coconut oil for few minutes, add all veggies and stir fry for 2 more minutes. Add the rest of the marinade and stir fry for a minute. Serve with brown rice or quinoa.

Zucchini, Shrimp, Red Pepper & Snow Peas Stir Fry

Serves 2

Ingredients - Allergies: SF, GF, DF, EF
- 1/2 pound shrimp • 1/2 cup sliced red peppers
- 1 cup sliced zucchini
- 1/2 cup broccoli
- 1 Tbsp. coconut oil

Instructions

Marinade shrimp in a Superfoods marinade. Stir fry drained shrimp in coconut oil for few minutes, add all veggies and stir fry for 2 more minutes. Add the rest of the marinade and stir fry for a minute. Serve with brown rice or quinoa.

Spicy Squid, Zucchini & Celery Stir Fry

Serves 2

Ingredients - Allergies: SF, GF, DF, EF
- 1/2 pound squid • 1/2 cup sliced zucchini
- 1 + 1/2 cup sliced celery
- 1/2 cup sliced onions
- 1 Tbsp. coconut oil
- 1 Tbsp. chili powder (to taste)

Instructions

Marinade squid in a Superfoods marinade. Stir fry drained squid in coconut oil for few minutes, add all veggies and stir fry for 2 more minutes. Add the rest of the marinade and stir fry for a minute. Serve with brown rice or quinoa.

Cabbage, Green Onions & Chicken Stir Fry

Serves 2

Ingredients - Allergies: SF, GF, DF, EF
- 1/2 pound sliced chicken • 1 cup sliced cabbage (or Chinese Napa cabbage)
- 1/2 cup sliced celery
- 2 sliced green onions
- 1/2 cup cashews
- 1 Tsp.oil *Instructions*

Marinade chicken in a Superfoods marinade. Stir fry drained chicken in coconut oil for few minutes, add all vegetables and stir fry for 2 more minutes. Add the rest of the marinade and stir fry for a minute. Serve with brown rice or quinoa.

Octopus, Green Peppers & Mushrooms Stir Fry

Serves 2

Ingredients - Allergies: SF, GF, DF, EF
- 1/2 pound cubed octopus • 1 cup sliced green peppers
- 1/2 cup sliced celery
- 1/2 cup sliced onions
- 1/2 cup sliced mushrooms
- 1 Tsp.oil *Instructions*

Marinade octopus in a Superfoods marinade. Stir fry drained octopus in coconut oil for few minutes, add all vegetables and stir fry for 2 more minutes. Add the rest of the marinade and stir fry for a minute. Serve with brown rice or quinoa.

Beef, Celery, Zucchini & Snow Peas Stir Fry

Serves 2

Ingredients - Allergies: SF, GF, DF, EF
- 1/2 pound cubed beef • 1 cup sliced zucchini
- 1/2 cup sliced celery
- 1/2 cup sliced onions
- 1/2 cup sliced snow peas
- 1 Tsp.oil *Instructions*

Marinade beef in a Superfoods marinade. Stir fry drained beef in coconut oil for few minutes, add all vegetables and stir fry for 2 more minutes. Add the rest of the marinade and stir fry for a minute. Serve with brown rice or quinoa.

Baby Octopus, Green Peppers & Carrot Stir Fry

Serves 2

Ingredients - Allergies: SF, GF, DF, EF
- 1/2 pound baby octopus • 1 cup sliced green peppers
- 1/2 cup sliced carrots
- 2 sliced green onions
- 1/2 cup cashews
- 1 Tsp.oil *Instructions*

Marinade octopus in a Superfoods marinade. Stir fry drained octopus in coconut oil for few minutes, add all vegetables and stir fry for 2 more minutes. Add the rest of the marinade and stir fry for a minute. Serve with brown rice or quinoa.

Naachi Bokum – Spicy Octopus Zucchini Stir Fry

Serves 2
Ingredients - Allergies: SF, GF, DF, EF
- 1/2 pound cubed octopus • 1 cup sliced zucchini
- 1/2 cup sliced carrot
- 2 sliced green onions
- 1/2 cup sliced celery
- 1 Tsp.oil and 1 tsp. chili *Instructions*

Marinade octopus in a Superfoods marinade and chili. Stir fry drained octopus in coconut oil for few minutes, add all vegetables and stir fry for 2 more minutes. Add the rest of the marinade and stir fry for a minute. Serve with brown rice or quinoa.

Beef, Zucchini & Yellow Peppers Stir Fry

Serves 2
Ingredients - Allergies: SF, GF, DF, EF
- 1/2 pound beef • 1 cup sliced zucchini
- 1 cup sliced yellow peppers
- 1/2 cup sliced Onions
- 1 Tbsp. oil *Instructions*

Marinade beef in a Superfoods marinade. Stir fry drained beef in coconut oil for few minutes, add all vegetables and stir fry for 2 more minutes. Add the rest of the marinade and stir fry for a minute. Serve with brown rice or quinoa.

Chicken, Green Beans & Broccoli Stir Fry

Serves 2
Ingredients - Allergies: SF, GF, DF, EF
- 1/2 pound chicken • 1 cup sliced green beans
- 1 cup sliced broccoli
- 1/2 cup sliced Onions
- 1 Tbsp. oil *Instructions*

Marinade chicken in a Superfoods marinade. Stir fry drained chicken in coconut oil for few minutes, add all vegetables and stir fry for 2 more minutes. Add the rest of the marinade and stir fry for a minute. Serve with brown rice or quinoa.

Pork, Onions & Celery on Lettuce Stir Fry

Serves 2

Ingredients - Allergies: SF, GF, DF, EF
- 1/2 pound pork, cubed • 2 cups sliced celery
- 1/2 cup sliced Onions
- 1 Tbsp. oil
- 2 cups lettuce leaves *Instructions*

Marinade pork in a Superfoods marinade. Stir fry drained pork in coconut oil for few minutes, add all vegetables and stir fry for 2 more minutes. Add the rest of the marinade and stir fry for a minute. Serve over lettuce leaves.

Chicken & Sprouts Stir Fry

Serves 2

Ingredients - Allergies: SF, GF, DF, EF
- 1/2 pound chicken • 2 cups sprouts
- 1 Tbsp. oil *Instructions*

Marinade chicken in a Superfoods marinade. Stir fry drained chicken in coconut oil for few minutes, add all vegetables and stir fry for 2 more minutes. Add the rest of the marinade and stir fry for a minute. Serve with brown rice or quinoa.

Chicken, Snow Peas & Mushrooms Stir Fry

Serves 2

Ingredients - Allergies: SF, GF, DF, EF
- 1/2 pound chicken • 1 cup sliced snow peas
- 1 cup sliced mushrooms
- 1/2 cup sliced Onions
- 1 Tbsp. oil *Instructions*

Marinade chicken in a Superfoods marinade. Stir fry drained chicken in coconut oil for few minutes, add all vegetables and stir fry for 2 more minutes. Add the rest of the marinade and stir fry for a minute. Serve with brown rice or quinoa.

Beef & Snow Peas Stir Fry

Serves 2

Ingredients - Allergies: SF, GF, DF, EF
- 1/2 pound beef • 2 cups sliced snow peas
- 1/2 cup sliced Onions
- 1 Tbsp. oil *Instructions*

Marinade beef in a Superfoods marinade. Stir fry drained beef in coconut oil for few minutes, add all vegetables and stir fry for 2 more minutes. Add the rest of the marinade and stir fry for a minute. Serve with brown rice or quinoa.

Chicken, Yellow Peppers & Green Beans Stir Fry

Serves 2

Ingredients - Allergies: SF, GF, DF, EF
- 1/2 pound chicken • 1 cup sliced green beans
- 1 cup sliced yellow peppers
- 1/2 cup sliced Onions
- 1 Tbsp. oil *Instructions*

Marinade chicken in a Superfoods marinade. Stir fry drained chicken in coconut oil for few minutes, add all vegetables and stir fry for 2 more minutes. Add the rest of the marinade and stir fry for a minute. Serve with brown rice or quinoa.

Shrimp, Broccoli, Carrot & Celery Stir Fry

Serves 2

Ingredients - Allergies: SF, GF, DF, EF
- 1/2 pound shrimp • 1 cup sliced Broccoli
- 1/2 cup sliced carrots
- 1/2 cup sliced celery
- 1/2 cup sliced Onions
- 1 Tbsp. oil *Instructions*

Marinade shrimp in a Superfoods marinade. Stir fry drained shrimp in coconut oil for few minutes, add all vegetables and stir fry for 2 more minutes. Add the rest of the marinade and stir fry for a minute. Serve with brown rice or quinoa.

Shrimp, Broccoli & Carrots Stir Fry

Serves 2

Ingredients - Allergies: SF, GF, DF, EF
- 1/2 pound shrimp • 1 cup sliced broccoli
- 1 cup sliced Carrots
- 1/2 cup sliced Onions
- 1 Tbsp. oil *Instructions*

Marinade shrimp in a Superfoods marinade. Stir fry drained shrimp in coconut oil for few minutes, add all vegetables and stir fry for 2 more minutes. Add the rest of the marinade and stir fry for a minute. Serve with brown rice or quinoa.

Chicken, Red Peppers & Green Peppers Stir Fry

Serves 2

Ingredients - Allergies: SF, GF, DF, EF
- 1/2 pound chicken • 1 cup sliced red peppers
- 1/2 cup sliced green peppers
- 1 cup sliced Onions
- 1 Tbsp. oil *Instructions*

Marinade chicken in a Superfoods marinade. Stir fry drained chicken in coconut oil for few minutes, add all vegetables and stir fry for 2 more minutes. Add the rest of the marinade and stir fry for a minute. Serve with brown rice or quinoa.

Beef, Chinese Cabbage & Carrots Stir Fry

Serves 2

Ingredients - Allergies: SF, GF, DF, EF
- 1/2 pound sliced beef • 1 cup sliced Chinese cabbage
- 2 cup julienned carrots
- 1/2 cup sliced Onions
- 1 Tbsp. oil *Instructions*

Marinade beef in a Superfoods marinade. Stir fry drained beef in coconut oil for few minutes, add all vegetables and stir fry for 2 more minutes. Add the rest of the marinade and stir fry for a minute. Serve with brown rice or quinoa.

Beef, Red Peppers & Asparagus Stir Fry

Serves 2

Ingredients - Allergies: SF, GF, DF, EF
- 1/2 pound beef • 1 cup sliced red peppers
- 1 cup sliced asparagus
- 1/2 cup sliced onions
- 1 Tbsp. oil *Instructions*

Marinade beef in a Superfoods marinade. Stir fry drained beef in coconut oil for few minutes, add all vegetables and stir fry for 2 more minutes. Add the rest of the marinade and stir fry for a minute. Serve with brown rice or quinoa.

Beef & Sugar Snap Peas Stir Fry

Serves 2

Ingredients - Allergies: SF, GF, DF, EF
- 1/2 pound beef • 2 cups sliced sugar snap peas
- 1 cup sliced Onions
- 1 Tbsp. oil *Instructions*

Marinade beef in a Superfoods marinade. Stir fry drained beef in coconut oil for few minutes, add all vegetables and stir fry for 2 more minutes. Add the rest of the marinade and stir fry for a minute. Serve with brown rice or quinoa.

Duck, Chinese Broccoli & Water Chestnut Stir Fry

Serves 2

Ingredients - Allergies: SF, GF, DF, EF
- 1/2 pound duck breast meat • 1 cup sliced Chinese broccoli
- 1/2 cup sliced Water Chestnut
- 1 cup sliced Onions
- 1 Tbsp. oil *Instructions*

Marinade duck in a Superfoods marinade. Stir fry drained duck in coconut oil for few minutes, add all vegetables and stir fry for 2 more minutes. Add the rest of the marinade and stir fry for a minute. Serve with brown rice or quinoa.

Shrimp, Long Beans & Pork Stir Fry

Serves 2

Ingredients - Allergies: SF, GF, DF, EF
- 1/4 pound pork • 1/4 pound shrimp
- 2 cups long beans
- 1/2 cup sliced Onions
- 1 Tbsp. oil *Instructions*

Marinade pork & shrimp in a Superfoods marinade. Stir fry drained pork & shrimp in coconut oil for few minutes, add all vegetables and stir fry for 2 more minutes. Add the rest of the marinade and stir fry for a minute. Serve with brown rice or quinoa.

Beef, Red Peppers & Eggplant Stir Fry

Serves 2

Ingredients - Allergies: SF, GF, DF, EF
- 1/2 pound beef • 1 cup sliced red peppers
- 1 cup Chinese eggplant
- 1/2 cup sliced Onions
- 1 Tbsp. oil *Instructions*

Marinade beef & eggplant in a Superfoods marinade. Stir fry drained beef and eggplant in coconut oil for few minutes, add all other vegetables and stir fry for 2 more minutes. Add the rest of the marinade and stir fry for a minute. Serve with brown rice or quinoa.

Duck, Fennel & Celery Stir Fry

Serves 2

Ingredients - Allergies: SF, GF, DF, EF
- 1/2 pound duck • 1 cup sliced celery
- 1 cup sliced fennel
- 1/2 cup sliced Onions
- 1 Tbsp. oil *Instructions*

Marinade duck in a Superfoods marinade. Stir fry drained duck in coconut oil for few minutes, add all vegetables and stir fry for 2 more minutes. Add the rest of the marinade and stir fry for a minute. Serve with brown rice or quinoa.

Squid, Okra & Kimchee Stir Fry

Serves 2

Ingredients - Allergies: SF, GF, DF, EF
- 1 cup okra • 1/2 pound Squid
- 1 cup kimchee
- 1/2 cup sliced Onions
- 1 Tbsp. oil *Instructions*

Marinade squid in a Superfoods marinade. Stir fry drained squid in coconut oil for few minutes, add all vegetables and stir fry for 2 more minutes. Add the rest of the marinade and stir fry for a minute. Serve with brown rice or quinoa.

Shrimp, Onions & Celery Stir Fry

Serves 2

Ingredients - Allergies: SF, GF, DF, EF
- 2 cups sliced celery • 1/2 pound shrimp
- 1/2 cup sliced Onions
- 1 Tbsp. oil *Instructions*

Marinade shrimp in a Superfoods marinade. Stir fry drained shrimp in coconut oil for few minutes, add all vegetables and stir fry for 2 more minutes. Add the rest of the marinade and stir fry for a minute. Serve with brown rice or quinoa.

Squid, Carrot, Red Peppers & Onion Stir Fry

Serves 2

Ingredients - Allergies: SF, GF, DF, EF
- 1 cup sliced carrot • 1/2 pound squid
- 1 cup sliced red peppers
- 1/2 cup sliced Onions
- 1 Tbsp. oil *Instructions*

Marinade squid in a Korean spicy Superfoods marinade. Stir fry drained squid in coconut oil for few minutes, add all vegetables and stir fry for 2 more minutes. Add the rest of the marinade and stir fry for a minute. Serve with brown rice or quinoa.

Beef, Carrot, Red Peppers & Green Onion Stir Fry

Serves 2

Ingredients - Allergies: SF, GF, DF, EF
- 1 sliced carrot • 1/2 pound beef
- 1 cup sliced red peppers
- 1 cup sliced green Onions
- 1 Tbsp. oil *Instructions*

Marinade beef in a Superfoods marinade. Stir fry drained beef in coconut oil for few minutes, add all vegetables and stir fry for 2 more minutes. Add the rest of the marinade and stir fry for a minute. Serve with brown rice or quinoa.

Mixed Seafood, Snow Peas & Celery Stir Fry

Serves 2

Ingredients - Allergies: SF, GF, DF, EF
- 1 sliced carrot • 1/2 pound mixed seafood
- 1 cup sliced snow peas
- 1 cup sliced celery
- 1/2 cup sliced Onions
- 1 Tbsp. oil *Instructions*

Marinade mixed seafood in Superfoods marinade. Stir fry drained mixed seafood in coconut oil for few minutes, add all vegetables and stir fry for 2 more minutes. Add the rest of the marinade and stir fry for a minute. Serve with brown rice or quinoa.

Pork, Carrot & Onion Stir Fry

Serves 2

Ingredients - Allergies: SF, GF, DF, EF
- 1 cup sliced carrot • 1/2 pound pork
- 1 cup sliced celery
- 1 cup sliced Onions
- 1 Tbsp. oil *Instructions*

Marinade pork in a Superfoods marinade. Stir fry drained pork in coconut oil for few minutes, add all vegetables and stir fry for 2 more minutes. Add the rest of the marinade and stir fry for a minute. Serve with brown rice or quinoa.

Shrimp, Corn & Leeks Stir Fry

Serves 2

Ingredients - Allergies: SF, GF, DF, EF
- 1 sliced carrot • 1/2 pound shrimp
- 1 cup drained corn
- 1 cup sliced Onions
- 1 Tbsp. oil *Instructions*

Marinade shrimp in Superfoods marinade. Stir fry drained shrimp in coconut oil for few minutes, add all vegetables and stir fry for 2 more minutes. Add the rest of the marinade and stir fry for a minute. Serve with brown rice or quinoa.

Squid, Green Peppers & Red Peppers Stir Fry

Serves 2

Ingredients - Allergies: SF, GF, DF, EF
- 1 cup sliced green peppers • 1/2 pound squid
- 1 cup sliced red peppers
- 1/2 cup sliced Onions
- 1 Tbsp. oil *Instructions*

Marinade squid in Superfoods marinade. Stir fry drained squid in coconut oil for few minutes, add all vegetables and stir fry for 2 more minutes. Add the rest of the marinade and stir fry for a minute. Serve with brown rice or quinoa.

Chickpeas, Zucchini & Chicken Stir Fry

Serves 2

Ingredients - Allergies: SF, GF, DF, EF
- 1 cup sliced green zucchini • 1/2 pound cooked and drained chickpeas
- 1 cup sliced yellow zucchini
- 1/2 cup sliced Onions
- 1 Tbsp. oil *Instructions*

Marinade chickpeas in Superfoods marinade. Stir fry drained chickpeas in coconut oil for few minutes, add all vegetables and stir fry for 2 more minutes. Add the rest of the marinade and stir fry for a minute. Serve with brown rice or quinoa.

Chinese Cabbage, Chicken, Carrot & Leeks Stir Fry

Serves 2

Ingredients - Allergies: SF, GF, DF, EF
- 1 cup sliced Chinese cabbage • 1/2 pound chicken
- 1 cup shredded carrot
- 1/2 cup sliced leeks
- 1 Tbsp. oil *Instructions*

Marinade chicken in Superfoods marinade. Stir fry drained chicken in coconut oil for few minutes, add all vegetables and stir fry for 2 more minutes. Add the rest of the marinade and stir fry for a minute. Serve with brown rice or quinoa.

Green Beans, Carrot, Red Peppers, Corn & Snow Peas Stir Fry

Serves 2

Ingredients - Allergies: SF, GF, DF, EF
- 1/2 cup sliced green beans
- 1/2 cup sliced snow peas • 1 cup cubed tofu
- 1/2 cup sliced red peppers
- 1/2 cup shredded carrots
- 1/2 cup corn
- 1/2 cup sliced Onions
- 1 Tbsp. oil *Instructions*

Marinade tofu in Superfoods marinade. Stir fry drained tofu in coconut oil for few minutes, add all vegetables and stir fry for 2 more minutes. Add the rest of the marinade and stir fry for a minute. Serve with brown rice or quinoa.

Pork, Zucchini, Red Pepper & Onion Stir Fry

Serves 2

Ingredients - Allergies: SF, GF, DF, EF
- 1 cup sliced zucchini • 1/2 pound pork
- 1 cup sliced red peppers
- 1/2 cup sliced Onions
- 1 Tbsp. oil *Instructions*

Marinade pork in Superfoods marinade. Stir fry drained pork in coconut oil for few minutes, add all vegetables and stir fry for 2 more minutes. Add the rest of the marinade and stir fry for a minute. Serve with brown rice or quinoa.

Shrimp, Carrot, Red Peppers & Green Onions Stir Fry

Serves 2

Ingredients - Allergies: SF, GF, DF, EF
- 1 cup sliced red peppers • 1/2 pound shrimp
- 1 cup shredded carrot
- 1/2 cup sliced green Onions
- 1 Tbsp. oil *Instructions*

Marinade shrimp in Superfoods marinade. Stir fry drained shrimp in coconut oil for few minutes, add all vegetables and stir fry for 2 more minutes. Add the rest of the marinade and stir fry for a minute. Serve with brown rice or quinoa.

Buddha's Delight Stir Fry

Serves 2
Ingredients - Allergies: SF, GF, DF, EF
- 1/2 cup sliced red peppers and fresh mushrooms each • 1/2 cup sliced bamboo shoots & green onions
- 1/2 cup shredded carrot & sliced snow peas, each
- 1/2 cup sprouts and pre-soaked dried mushrooms
- 1 Tbsp. oil *Instructions*

Marinade all mushrooms in Superfoods marinade. Stir fry drained mushrooms in coconut oil for few minutes, add all vegetables and stir fry for 2 more minutes. Add the rest of the marinade and stir fry for a minute. Serve with brown rice or quinoa.

Chicken, Chinese Cabbage & Mushrooms Stir Fry

Serves 2
Ingredients - Allergies: SF, GF, DF, EF
- 1 cup sliced Chinese Cabbage • 1/2 pound chicken
- 1 cup sliced mushrooms
- 1/2 cup sliced green Onions
- 1 Tbsp. oil *Instructions*

Marinade chicken in Superfoods marinade. Stir fry drained chicken in coconut oil for few minutes, add all vegetables and stir fry for 2 more minutes. Add the rest of the marinade and stir fry for a minute. Serve with brown rice or quinoa.

Chicken, Mushrooms & Leeks Stir Fry

Serves 2
Ingredients - Allergies: SF, GF, DF, EF
- 1 cup sliced leeks • 1/2 pound chicken
- 1 cup sliced mushrooms
- 1/2 cup shredded carrots
- 1 Tbsp. oil *Instructions*

Marinade chicken in Superfoods marinade. Stir fry drained chicken in coconut oil for few minutes, add all vegetables and stir fry for 2 more minutes. Add the rest of the marinade and stir fry for a minute. Serve with brown rice or quinoa.

Chicken, Walnuts & Mushrooms Stir Fry

Serves 2

Ingredients - Allergies: SF, GF, DF, EF
- 2 cups sliced Mushrooms • 1/2 pound chicken
- 1/2 cup walnuts
- 1/2 cup sliced green Onions
- 1 Tbsp. oil *Instructions*

Marinade chicken in Superfoods marinade. Stir fry drained chicken in coconut oil for few minutes, add all vegetables and stir fry for 2 more minutes. Add the rest of the marinade and stir fry for a minute. Serve with brown rice or quinoa.

Venison Szechuan Stir Fry

Serves 2

Ingredients - Allergies: SF, GF, DF, EF
- 2 cups sliced red peppers • 1/2 pound venison meat
- 1/2 cup sliced leeks
- 1 Tbsp. oil

Instructions

Marinade venison in Superfoods marinade. Stir fry drained venison in coconut oil for few minutes, add all vegetables and stir fry for 2 more minutes. Add the rest of the marinade and stir fry for a minute. Serve with brown rice or quinoa.

Mushrooms, Pork, Green Beans & Carrot Stir Fry

Serves 2

Ingredients - Allergies: SF, GF, DF, EF
- 2 cups sliced mushrooms • 1/2 pound pork meat
- 1/2 cup sliced green beans
- 1/2 cup sliced carrots
- 1/2 cup sliced red peppers
- 1 Tbsp. oil

Instructions

Marinade pork in Superfoods marinade. Stir fry drained pork in coconut oil for few minutes, add all vegetables and stir fry for 2 more minutes. Add the rest of the marinade and stir fry for a minute. Serve with brown rice or quinoa.

Red & Green Peppers, Eggplant & Leeks Stir Fry

Serves 2

Ingredients - Allergies: SF, GF, DF, EF
- 2 cups sliced red & green peppers • 1 large eggplant, cubed
- 1/2 cup sliced leeks
- 1 Tbsp. oil

Instructions

Marinade eggplant in Superfoods marinade. Stir fry drained eggplant in coconut oil for few minutes, add all vegetables and stir fry for 2 more minutes. Add the rest of the marinade and stir fry for a minute. Serve with brown rice or quinoa.

Red Peppers, Leeks & Chicken Stir Fry

Serves 2

Ingredients - Allergies: SF, GF, DF, EF
- 2 cups sliced red peppers • 1/2 pound chicken meat
- 1/2 cup sliced leeks
- 1 Tbsp. oil

Instructions

Marinade chicken in Superfoods marinade. Stir fry drained chicken in coconut oil for few minutes, add all vegetables and stir fry for 2 more minutes. Add the rest of the marinade and stir fry for a minute. Serve with brown rice or quinoa.

Shiitake, Sprouts, Snow Peas & Carrots Stir Fry

Serves 2

Ingredients - Allergies: SF, GF, DF, EF
- 1 cup sliced shiitake • 1 cup sprouts
- 1/2 cup sliced snow peas
- 1/2 cup sliced carrots
- 1/2 cup sliced yellow peppers
- 1 Tbsp. oil

Instructions

Marinade shiitake in Superfoods marinade. Stir fry drained shiitake in coconut oil for few minutes, add all vegetables and stir fry for 2 more minutes. Add the rest of the marinade and stir fry for a minute. Serve with brown rice or quinoa.

Turkey, Red & Yellow Peppers, Broccoli Stir Fry

Serves 2

Ingredients - Allergies: SF, GF, DF, EF
- 2 cups sliced red peppers • 1/2 pound turkey meat
- 1/2 cup sliced broccoli
- 1/2 cup sliced yellow peppers
- 1/2 cup sliced red peppers
- 1/2 cup julienned zucchini
- 1 Tbsp. oil

Instructions

Marinade turkey in Superfoods marinade. Stir fry drained turkey in coconut oil for few minutes, add all vegetables and stir fry for 2 more minutes. Add the rest of the marinade and stir fry for a minute. Serve with brown rice or quinoa.

CPSIA information can be obtained
at www.ICGtesting.com
Printed in the USA
LVHW061257190222
711186LV00026B/560

9 781649 849175